"With his extensive clinical experience, Dr. Rundbaken has done a good job of presenting the complex world of valley fever. I recommend this book to patients, medical students and physicians."

— AMARDEEP MAJHAIL

"This book is a captivating portrait of valley fever. It is well written, carefully researched and very informative. I highly recommend it to everyone: patients, medical personel and epidemiologists."

— MANDEEP K. RAI

"This book provides both patient and provider a concise and thorough summary of valley fever and why everyone should pay attention to this potentially devastating illness."

—ANNE GERTH, R.N., GNP-C

"I personally experienced Dr. Rundbaken's expertise during my yearlong battle with valley fever. I believe that information is the key to personal health This book provides it!"

—BRIAN MURPHY

"Misdiagnosed five times, I was referred to Dr. Rundbaken and learned I had valley fever meningitis. He saved my life! This book is for anyone concerned about diagnosis and treatment"

—JAMIE HUTH

"My job involves seeing the devastation of valley fever in patients … and then a relief from suffering. The disease is explained here in terms that everyone can understand."

—JUDY FOSKETT,
MEDICAL OFFICE MANAGER

VALLEY FEVER
Silent Epidemic

The Common, Often
Misdiagnosed Desert Ailment

Craig Rundbaken, D.O.

Valley Fever Silent Epidemic
Craig Rundbaken, D.O.

All rights reserved. No part of this publication may be transmitted or reproduced in any media or form without the express consent of the author.

Copyright © 2014 Craig Rundbaken, D.O.

ISBN 978-0-9907105-0-9

Printed in the USA by MiniBük

ACKNOWLEDGEMENTS

THIS BOOK WAS MADE POSSIBLE thanks to the help of several people. Thanks to my wife, Laura, and my daughter Ariel for their support in reviewing this manuscript and for being such important people in my life.

Thanks to David Seid and Kee Rash of Access Laser Press and to editors Mary L. Holden, and Hal DeKeyser and to Theresa Hunt, who provided transcription.

Thanks to Garry Cole, Ph.D., John Galgiani, M.D., Amardeep Majhail, M.D., Mandeep Rai M.D., Ann Gerth, N.P., Heather Smith M.D., Patricia White, David Bartsch Information Technology support-always a bullseye and Judy Foskett, my office manager, for reviewing the manuscript and providing helpful comments and direction. Clarisse A. Tsang, MPH, Senior Epidemiologist at the Arizona Department of Health Services was very helpful in reviewing the manuscript and allowing use of data and graphs from the Valley Fever 2012 Annual Report.

Case reporting by providers and laboratories is the key to Arizona's infectious disease surveillance system. All staff within the ADHS Office of Infectious Disease Services and local health departments are acknowledged for their contributions to data collection, data entry and data analysis. Funds and technical assistance from the Arizona Biomedical Research Commission (ABRC), the Centers for Disease Control and Prevention (CDC), and the University of Arizona Valley Fever Center for Excellence (VFCE) supported this work. The contents of this report are solely the responsibility of the authors and do not represent the official views of the ABRC, rhe CDC, or the VFCE.

TABLE OF CONTENTS

Introduction from the Author ix

Chapter 1 – An Overview of Valley Fever 1

Chapter 2 – Valley Fever Center for Excellence. 7

Chapter 3 – Contracting the Valley Fever Illness. 9

Chapter 4 – Valley Fever's Common Symptoms 13

Chapter 5 – Clinical Clues and Signs of Valley Fever. . 17

Chapter 6 – Laboratory Diagnosis of Valley Fever. . . . 25

Chapter 7 – Valley Fever and the Lungs, Plus Some Interesting Facts. 33

Chapter 8 – Valley Fever: Up Close and Personal 41

Chapter 9 – Treatment of Valley Fever 53

Chapter 10 – Risk Groups. 69

Chapter 11 – Case Rates and Epidemiology 73

Chapter 12 – Clinical Perspectives. 83

Chapter 13 – Prevention of Valley Fever 87

Chapter 14 – Valley Fever in Dogs 91

Chapter 15 – The Economic Impact of Valley Fever . . 93

Chapter 16 – Fast Fascinating Facts and Resource. . . 101

Resources. 107

Bibliography 109

Glossary. 123

INTRODUCTION FROM THE AUTHOR

OFTEN IN MEDICINE there are exact health problems with exact solutions. For example, a diseased gallbladder needs surgical removal. A woman in labor needs the baby delivered. A hip fractured in a fall needs repair by an orthopedic surgeon. This is the story of a disease that puzzles even the best clinicians.

That disease is valley fever.

What is valley fever? The purpose of this book is to answer that question. I want to clarify this illness to create more accuracy and efficiency in diagnosis and treatment. My goal is to raise awareness so people who are not health care professionals can prompt friends and family to seek medical attention and request examination and testing if signs and symptoms of valley fever occur. While this may read like a thesis—footnotes show the research—it is meant to be a resource for physicians and medical professionals as well as patients. A lot of research has been done; more is needed and everyone needs to care about it.

Do you know someone who went to the emergency room or saw a doctor to get a diagnosis for a respiratory ailment and a prescription for an antibiotic cure? If the antibiotic worked—fine. But if it didn't, there were probably more antibiotics prescribed. The respiratory ailment could have been valley fever. Valley fever does not respond to antibiotics. Perhaps the health professional did diagnose valley fever but said, "We do not need to treat it. It will resolve on its own."

The blood tests for valley fever can be false positive as well as false negative (Kuberski T, Herrig J, Pappagianis D, 2010) (Pappagianis D, Zimmer BL, 1990) (Sobonya R, Barbee RA, Wiens J, Trego D, 1990). The Arizona Department of Health Services requires all positive results for the disease to be reported and then be included in its statistics, thus using the data to track the disease.

Because valley fever can appear clinically similar to other diseases, patients are often misdiagnosed. A valley fever patient appeared to have an allergic reaction—a rash—and was treated with steroids. But steroids can worsen valley fever. Highly educated, well-trained physicians gave another valley fever victim, a hospitalized patient who was labeled with acute systemic lupus, high doses of the medications steroids and methotrexate. The patient died of complications of valley fever, yet she was only in her early 40s. There are many examples of delayed and missed diagnosis of valley fever—due to its variable and enigmatic clinical course as well as the mobility of our society—people traveling from endemic to non-endemic regions (where the disease is often not considered in a diagnosis).

In addition, the endemic region for the *cocci* spores that cause valley fever may have been underestimated. Recent cases in south central Washington have been diagnosed and there has been soil culture confirmation of the fungal spores. This is a region not before known to harbor the fungi. (MMWR 2014 May 23; 63(20):450. Marsden-Haug, N. et al)

One group of doctors says they treat and prescribe medication for all patients diagnosed with valley fever because it could spread or worsen. However, some research studies showed that patients who were given treatment for the disease were worse off than those who went untreated with antifungal therapy while still under medical care. Because of this conundrum, doctors face legal implications. They will be sued for malpractice and asked during depositions, "Why did you withhold treatment?"

Further confounding the clinical course of valley fever cases, medical imaging reports often convey the lung abnormalities for valley fever, which is consistent with metastatic cancer leading to a computed tomography (CT) scan, or a positron emission tomography (PET) scan and a subsequent lung biopsy, raising the cost of misdiagnosis. Most doctors agree that a biopsy must be done if cancer is suspected—especially if patient has risk factors such as being a smoker—although many cases turn out to be valley fever tumors, nodules or abscesses.

The experienced clinician wants to wait and follow the patient in the office, through check-ups. What if the patient has lung cancer and not valley fever—or both? I've seen this diagnostic situation of combined disease several times. This also can present treatment dilemmas for oncologists and radiation oncologists trying to determine what is cancer or infection in the lung or other organs.

Here's another misdiagnosis scenario to consider. A seasonal visitor to Arizona goes home for Christmas to Washington and a few days later falls gravely ill, on life support, diagnosed with pneumonia. His wife asks that the Washington physician consider valley fever fungal pneumonia instead of bacterial pneumonia. She calls an Arizona doctor in a panic and says she is being ignored. Her husband slowly improved and weeks later he returned to Arizona where he was evaluated and his lab results were positive for valley fever. He was prescribed antifungal therapy for persistent lingering symptoms and to relieve anxiety that he was not treated for his cocci infection and slowly resolved his illness over the next few weeks.

The mystery that surrounds valley fever is astounding. A colleague of mine went to a seminar on valley fever and told me he had more questions after it than before—many diagnostic tests are ambiguous. He compared valley fever to other diseases in his practice such as diabetes, hypertension or lipid management where a lack of definitive diagnostic tests creates risk for the patient and liability to his practice.

One of the reasons for such confusion can be seen in the following case history: Janice, a 35-year-old woman, moved to Arizona because the Minnesota winters were hard on her—she suffered with rheumatoid arthritis. She became even sicker after her move to Surprise, a Phoenix suburb. She'd been using the immunosuppressive medications prednisone, methotrexate and Remicade, and within two weeks she'd developed pneumonia and severe headaches. The diagnosis was made for valley fever pneumonia and valley fever meningitis after having seen several doctors and multiple antibiotics. As her initial presentation appeared similar to bronchitis or a viral infection, the diagnosis was not made or considered.

She was happy with her move to Arizona but felt dismayed there were no governmental or public service messages about valley fever that told her that her new home in a dusty construction zone created a risk of infection. Frustration and disappointment in learning that many people refer to valley fever as Arizona's little secret has caused Janice's condition to worsen—not improve. Subsequently, she was placed on medical disability and continues on 600 mg a day of fluconazole.

Fortunately, most people who contract valley fever overcome it with no long term related health issues and are immune protected from it. However, achieving a diagnosis can be a complex process and often requires experienced clinicians in the endemic area.

What's up with this illness, valley fever? A mystery illness that puzzled so many physicians at the turn of the 20th century continues to confuse even experienced physicians. There are persistent efforts to ring the alarms about valley fever by a relatively small group and continued disappointment that our government leaders have not encouraged a herculean effort to finally get a drug that will kill the fungus or a vaccine to prevent it.

In this book you will read all I have to offer about valley fever—science, treatment options and resources available to help those suffering with the disease find relief and return to good health.

CRAIG M. RUNDBAKEN, D.O., FACOI, FCCP, is board certified in Internal Medicine, Pulmonary Disease and Sleep Medicine. He is a fellow of the American College of Osteopathic Internists, as well as the College of Chest Physicians. He is a 1992 medical graduate of Des Moines University and 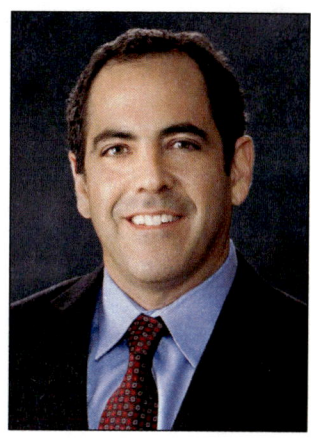 completed a residency in internal medicine at Garden City Hospital in conjunction with Michigan State University in 1995. His pulmonary fellowship was completed in 1997 at Botsford General Hospital in Farmington Hills, Michigan.

Dr. Rundbaken received a B.S. in Psychology from the University of Wisconsin, Whitewater in 1986. Practicing in Arizona since 1997, Dr. Rundbaken's office is at 13949 W. Meeker Blvd., Suite D, Sun City West, AZ 85375—The Respiratory and Valley Fever Clinic.

He founded the Respiratory and Valley Fever Clinic in 2003 after diagnosing and treating many valley fever patients. He is one of the founding board members of Valley Fever Alliance of Arizona Clinicians, associated with the University of Arizona. In 2011, Dr. Rundbaken became a board member of Arizona Victims of Valley Fever, Inc., founded by Patricia White. Its goal is to promote education, awareness and cure.

Dr. Rundbaken is also medical director at Goodnight Sleep Lab, with three locations in the Phoenix metropolitan area. He has hospital privileges at Banner Del E. Webb Memorial Hospital, Banner Boswell Medical Center and Banner Thunderbird Medical Center.

CHAPTER 1

An Overview of Valley Fever

VALLEY FEVER CAN STRIKE ANYONE, at any time, and create long-lasting health issues. Here is another example of how valley fever runs its course:

Ryan was a 35-year-old executive who loved riding his quad (all-terrain vehicle) through the Sonoran Desert. Three weeks after a particularly dusty ride, he went to his doctor feeling extreme fatigue, weakness, coughing, congested and experiencing a 15-pound weight loss. He was diagnosed with pneumonia but despite antibiotics still felt unusually tired and unable to work.

After seeing a specialist, a CT chest scan demonstrated large lymph nodes in his chest and a possible tumor. The valley fever antibodies that showed up in his lab work were positive. Due to concern about simultaneous lymphoma and valley fever, a lymph node biopsy was performed. No cancer was seen, but he developed a rare complication of chylothorax (thoracic duct tear causing chylous fluid build-up in pleural space within the chest cavity) and required lung surgery and prolonged hospitalization.

Post-discharge and three-month recuperation, he returned to work but required a year of antifungal treatment before feeling entirely recovered.

Valley fever is a term to describe the constellation of physical symptoms caused by the soil fungus called *Coccidioides*. Two species have been identified in the genus: *Coccidioides immitis*, which was originally identified in California and more recently, *Coccidioides posadasii*, which is more common in Arizona. These fungi are commonly known as *cocci*. The first known case was an Argentinean soldier, Domingo Ezcurra, in 1893. He was treated in a Buenos Aires hospital after developing disfiguring facial lesions and a constellation of other symptoms, including fever, rash, swollen lymph nodes, etc. The biopsied lesions were puzzling; they were attributed to a protozoan that resembled an organism that infected chickens. In 1900, W. Ophuls, M.D. correctly identified fungal spore and mycelium. (Ophuls W, Moffitt HC, 1900) (Fisher MC, Koenig GL, White TJ, Taylor JW, 2002) Experts had identified the diagnostic confusion between the protozoan and the fungus, but the link between the fungus and an escalating valley fever epidemic in the San Joaquin Valley did not occur until over 30 years later.

Cocci is common in Arizona's desert, particularly in the counties of Maricopa (Phoenix and suburbs, known as the Valley of the Sun), Pima (Tucson) and Pinal (Casa

Grande). In California, *cocci* is common. Kern County, and in particular the San Joaquin Valley (including Bakersfield and Modesto), are places where valley fever cases are highly concentrated. (California Department of Public Health. Coccidioidomycosis yearly summary report 2001 – 2010) (Increase in reported coccidioidomycosis – United States 1998-2011, 2013) (Sunenshine RH, Anderson, Erhart L, et al., 2007) (Arizona Department of Public Health)

The link between the infecting fungus and valley fever illness was not identified until a medical student named Harold Chope, who was working in the laboratory of Ernest C. Dickson, M.D. at Stanford medical school, was infected after accidently inhaling spores of *Coccidioides* from an open Petri dish on August 28, 1929. Nine days later, Chope became very ill with fever, chills, sweats and pneumonia with erythema nodosum (inflammation of the skin on his legs). Dr. Dickson later recognized Chope's illness as similar to the illnesses seen in the growing agriculture and cattle ranching industry in San Joaquin Valley referred to as San Joaquin Valley Fever. (Valley Fever of the San Joaquin Valley and the fungus Coccidioides, 1937)

After other cases were identified, working with Dr. Myrnie Gifford, M.D. at the Kern county health department, a paper was published in *Cal West Medicine* (1937 September; 47(3) 151-155), "Valley Fever of the San Joaquin Valley and the Fungus Coccidioides."

Despite the unraveling of the valley fever mystery, the disease can still be quite enigmatic and diagnosis can be delayed or completely missed. Over 77 years since the recognition of the causative agent for valley fever, no specific *Coccidioides*-targeted antifungal medication has been developed to treat valley fever, and no vaccine exists.

Valley fever has been known by many names through the decades, but health professionals refer to valley fever's causative agent as *cocci*, short for *Coccidioides*, and to valley fever as *coccidioidomycosis*. So, the terms *cocci* and valley fever are synonymous.

Here is the list of terms for valley fever: *cocci* (pronounced as "coxie"), desert fever, desert rheumatism (because it includes arthritis symptoms), San Joaquin Valley Fever and Wernicke-Posadasii disease, named for the two physicians who worked with the first known case in Buenos Aires. (Deresinski, 1980) (Dismukes WE, Pappas PG, Sobel JD, 2003) (Drutz DJ, Catanzaro A, 1978) (Drutz DJ, Catanzaro A, 1978) (Galgiani JN, et al) (Galgiani, Coccidioidomycosis: A regional disease of national importance, an update.Rethinking, 1999)

As a pulmonologist practicing at a Mecca for this disease, I have witnessed significant morbidity and occasional death from valley fever. *Cocci* can be difficult to diagnose as it presents much like any other respiratory infection. When visitors to Arizona arrive home and become ill, valley fever is often not considered. It can be argued that valley fever, relative to other diseases, has been minimized and trivialized.

It's time for new light to be shown on the disease of valley fever.

CHAPTER 2

Valley Fever Center for Excellence

IN 1996, VALLEY FEVER CENTER FOR EXCELLENCE started through the University of Arizona under John N. Galgiani, M.D. Its stated mission is to raise awareness and facilitate medical care for valley fever. Dr. Galgiani and his staff have been a resource for physicians and patients in Arizona and throughout the world. A significant amount of information is on the website: www.VFCE.arizona.edu/

In 2009, the Valley Fever Corridor Project, along with the Valley Fever Alliance of Arizona Clinicians (VFAAC), was formed upon recognition that the majority of valley fever cases are in the I-10 corridor between Phoenix and Tucson in Maricopa, Pima and Pinal counties. Physicians are encouraged to attend continuing medical education courses and become members. Members can obtain other medical specialty expertise through a password-protected website. The collaboration between researchers and physicians in the Corridor Project and the VFAAC will improve communication and treatment plans. This will also provide a reservoir of physicians and patients who can take part in medical studies (such as future vaccine studies and clinical trials of the drug Nikkomycin-z).

Clinicians interested in becoming members should contact the Valley Fever Center for Excellence at MDTC-VFAAC@email.arizona.edu.

CHAPTER 3

Contracting the Valley Fever Illness

THE SOURCE OF INFECTION, called the arthrospore, exists as a mycelium (mold) on the soil's surface, typically to a depth of six inches. Branching filamentous hyphae with alternating live barrel-shaped arthrospores are connected by a disjuncture cell. Disturbance of the soil sends the spores flying into the air. (Tamerius JD, Comrie DC, 2011) (Laniado-Laborin, 2007) (Saubolle MA, McKellar PP, Sussland D, 2007) (Pappagianis, Epidemiology of Coccidioidomycosis, 1988)

Valley fever infection and transmission usually occurs only when a human or animal inhales the desert soil fungal spore. Very rarely is there direct inoculation from a puncture wound or animal-caused infection; however, there has been a reported case of a cat bite transmission. (Gaidici A, Saubolle MA, 2009)

Cocci are described as dimorphic because once inhaled into the lung, the spore begins to change form. Over the next 72 hours, the endospore (a cylindrical-shaped arthrospore) enlarges from 3 – 5 micrometers to

75 micrometers and forms a round cell referred to as a spherule. The spherule becomes compartmentalized by internal septation and the compartments differentiate into a multitude of endospores. The spherule enlarges as the endospores mature, and then the released endospores infect nearby tissues. This cycle may repeat. The endospores may travel through the blood (known as hematogenous transfer) or through the lymphatic system to other organs. (Valley Fever Center for Excellence) (Drutz DJ, Catanzaro A, 1978) (Drutz DJ, Catanzaro A, 1978) (Hedges E, Miller S., 1990) (Hospenthal, 2013) (Stevens, 1995) (Sun SH, Huppert M, 1976) (Cole GT, Sun SH, 1985)

Valley fever is not contagious person-to-person.

Once arthrospores are inhaled from the environment, about 40 percent of people will become symptomatic while 60 percent develop minimal symptoms or none at all. Typically the symptoms occur within one to four weeks. (Palmer CE, Edwards PQ, Alfather WE, 1957) (Pappagianis, Epidimiology of Coccidioidomycosis Infection. 1988) (Saubolle MA, McKellar PP, Sussland D, 2007) (Smith CE, Beard RR, 1946) (Valley Fever Center of Excellence) (Galgiani, Coccidioidomycosis: A regional disease of national importance, an update. Rethinking, 1999)

A person's individual exposure to the arthrospore, or a large inoculum of arthrospores, as well as their health history, age, race, sex and immune status all factor into

The Morphology of Coccidioides

The soil phase or saprophytic cycle on left then the disturbed spore gets inhaled starting the parasitic cycle.

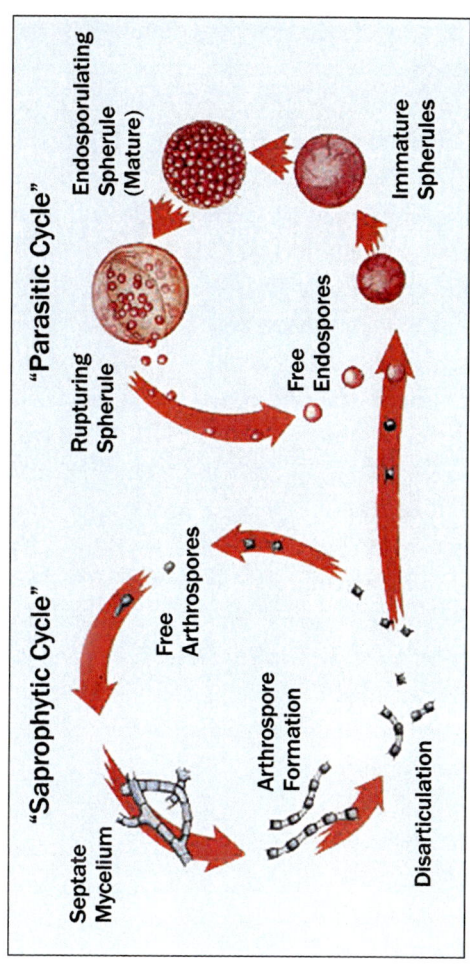

With permission from D. Hillel, B. Levine

the severity of their valley fever illness. Risk groups are described in Chapter 7. Paradoxically, the worst cases of valley fever usually befall otherwise normal, healthy people.

The amount of arthrospores an individual inhales may directly correlate with the severity of infection. For example, on June 19, 2001 at Dinosaur National Monument on the border of Colorado and Utah, all 10 of a group of archeological workers became ill with valley fever after laying stones, building a retaining wall and sifting for artifacts. This demonstrates a significant exposure and also the adaptability and the hardiness of this fungus as these cases were presumably outside the typical endemic zone. (Peterson LR, Marshall SL, Barton-Dixon C, Hajjeh RA, et al, Coccidioidomycosis among workers at an archaeological site, Northeastern Utah. Journal of Emerging Infectious Disease, 10 (4))

From September 10 to October 27, 2001, 23 Navy SEALs training in the San Joaquin Valley for six weeks were afflicted with valley fever. Ten of the 22 men who were evaluated had serological (blood test) evidence of valley fever. This represents 45 percent of the SEALs, the highest reported rate of valley fever ever to this military unit during field training. (Crum N, Lamb C, Utz G, Amundson D, Wallace M, 2002)

A large inoculum in outbreaks such as these can cause serious illness, but most infections are thought to be from a single spore or very low inoculums.

CHAPTER 4

Valley Fever's Common Symptoms

PEOPLE WHO GET VALLEY FEVER can be difficult to diagnose in the endemic region but when visitors to these areas return home to other states and countries, the illness can be quite perplexing to health care providers unfamiliar with the way it presents. Patients are typically given antibiotics when an antifungal medication is required. One study demonstrated that 29 percent of pneumonia in the endemic region had *cocci* pneumonia and was not bacterial or viral. (Valdivia L, Nix D, Wright M, Lindberg E, Fagan T, Lieberman D, et al, 2006)

Based on skin tests through epidemiological studies dating back to the 1940s and 1950s led by Charles Smith, M.D., 60 percent of patients who contracted valley fever did not have any symptoms, and 40 percent had mild to severe symptoms. (Smith CE, Whiting EG, Baker EE, Rosenberger HG, Beard RR, Saito MT, 1948) (Palmer CE, Edwards PQ, Alfather WE, 1957)

In 2007, the Arizona Department of Health Services interviewed 493 patients with valley fever. Below is a list of the greatest reported symptoms to the least. Note that 3 percent of those diagnosed with valley fever reported no symptoms. All figures represent a percentage of 100. (Arizona Department of Health Services, Valley Fever Report. May 2008)

- Fatigue – 84.4
- Cough – 66.9 *DRY*
- Shortness of breath – 58.7
- Fever – 54.1
- Night sweats – 52.0
- Chest pain – 48.8
- Chills – 47.8
- Joint pain – 47.2 *left leg*
- Headaches – 42.45 *2 days*
- Muscle pain – 41.1
- Wheezing – 37.4
- Rash – 33.9
- Stiff neck – 29.45
- Sore throat – 27.9
- Weight loss – 24.6
- Coughing up blood – 9.2 *1 day*

Fatigue is the most profound symptom for most patients. Many people feel tired, weak and unable to perform their typical work schedule. The Arizona Department of

Health Services study data (TsangCA, Anderson SM. Imholte SB, Erhart LM, et al. Enhanced surveillance of coccidioidomycosis. Arizona, USA 2007-2008. Emerging Infectious Diseases. 2010:16(11): 1738-44) on the impact of valley fever symptoms in peoples' lives is consistent with my personal experience caring for valley fever patients in Sun City West, Arizona:

- Patients were sick with valley fever for greater than six months (median 120 days)
- 74 percent of patients missed work due to *cocci* an average of one month (median 14 days)
- 75 percent were unable to do their usual activities for more than three months (median 47 days)

In summary, symptoms vary and it is important that healthcare professionals take into account the patient's travel history in considering a diagnosis of valley fever. Even brief exposures to wind-driven arthrospores while driving through an endemic zone, changing planes and even attending or participating in a sporting event can result in *cocci* exposure and cause an individual to contract valley fever.

CHAPTER 5

Clinical Clues and Signs of Valley Fever

APPROXIMATELY 25% OR LESS of patients will develop a skin rash. A variety of rashes are known to occur. Joint pain is another common symptom. Here are other symptoms medical professionals may find: (FieseMJ. Coccidioidomyosis.Springfield IL: Charles C. Thomas, 1958). (Drutz DJ, Catanzaro A, 1978)

Toxic erythema. This is a fine, red, diffuse rash that may resemble the measles and is commonly associated with fever. It dissipates in about one week. (Dismukes WE, Pappas PG, Sobel JD, 2003) (Kirkland TN, Fierer J., 1996) (Stevens, 1995)

Erythema nodosum. This is another common rash, which is felt to be a hypersensitivity type of reaction (allergic). It is more common in females. It has several qualities:

- Painful, red nodules below the skin along the anterior shins
- This rash is considered to be a good sign as it is associated with the development of cellular immune response and production of antibodies to combat the infection

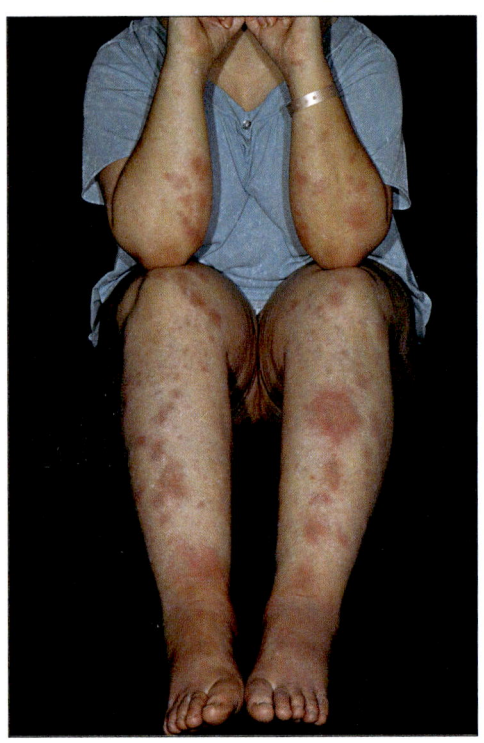

It is important to note that other illnesses can cause erythema nodosum. Other illnesses that cause erythema nodosum include tuberculosis, sarcoidosis, drug reactions including to sulfa, and bacterial streptococcal infections.

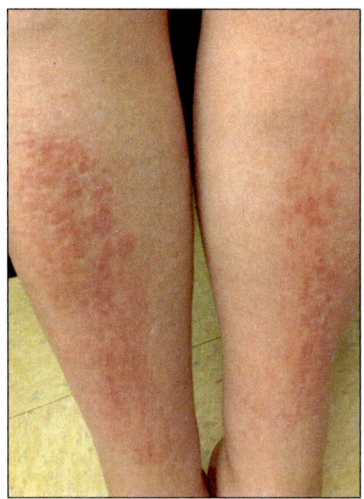

Erythema nodosum

- Lesions regress in approximately one to two weeks and may leave a pigment on the skin that slowly fades over a few weeks

Erythema multiforme. As with erythema nodosum, erythema multiforme can also be seen with other infections, drug reactions and diseases. Its symptoms are:

- Red, target-shaped crops of skin lesions
- Can be very itchy
- Common on the upper body

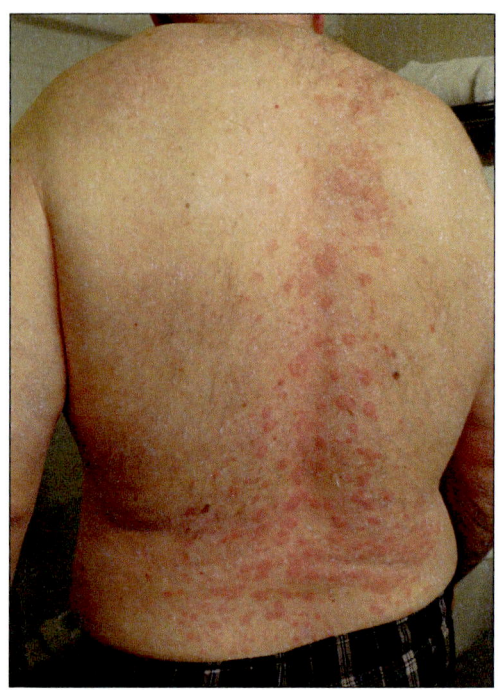

Erythema multiforme

- Common to the inner thighs
- It is an allergic type of hypersensitivity reaction to the fungus
- May have blisters or vesicles
- Can be like hives

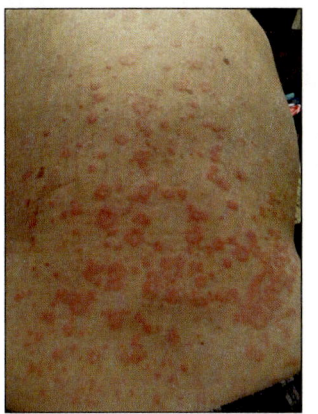 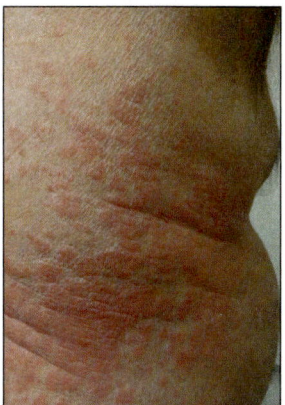

Left: Erythema multiform target red lesions back. Right: Erythema multiform right posterior flank.

The above rashes are not caused by the fungus spreading to the skin but are considered hypersensitive reactions to the fungus. When the fungus spreads to the skin or other organs, it is called disseminated disease.

Always biopsy a rash that fails to resolve

Disseminated skin lesions. Spread from the lung through the blood or the lymph system to the skin, these lesions have no particular predilection but can arise in areas where previous trauma has occurred. It is important that health professional's biopsy a skin rash that is not

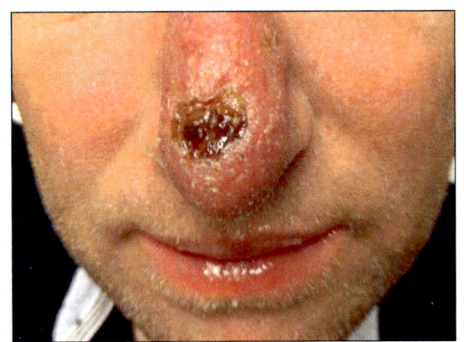

Cocci disseminated to the nose.

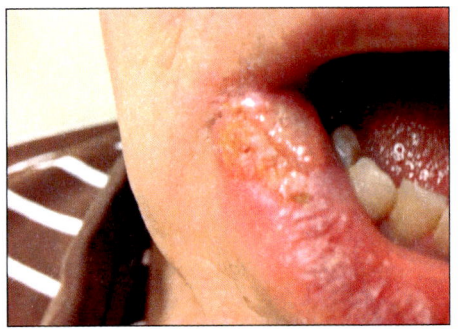

Cocci dissemination to right lower lip.

improving to assess for infectious *Coccidioides* or other causes such as skin cancer, allergies or drug reactions.

Patients who go to the emergency department or urgent care with a rash are treated with medications such as corticosteroids and antihistamines for an allergic reaction when the underlying problem might be *coccidioidomycosis*. It is important that valley fever be considered as corticosteroids can worsen *Coccidioides* and *coccidioidomycosis* infections.

Desert rheumatism. Arthritis-type pains may be associated with valley fever infections (known as primary pulmonary *coccidioidomycosis*). Here is information on the symptoms of this kind of pain, also known as desert rheumatism:

- Often seen with erythema nodosum
- Pain in the ankles, knees and wrists is common
- Joint pain is felt to be immune-related, not disseminated disease (spread outside the lung)

(Galgiani JN, et al) (Galgiani, Coccidioidomycosis: A regional disease of national importance, an update. Rethinking, 1999) (Drutz DJ, Catanzaro A, 1978) (Drutz DJ, Catanzaro A, 1978) (Brown J, Benedict K, Park BJ, Thompson III, GR, 2013) (Valley Fever Center of Excellence) (Deresinski, 1980) (Hospenthal, 2013) (Kirkland TN, Fierer J., 1996) (Pappagianis, Epidimiology of Coccidioidomycosis infection. 1988) (Stevens, 1995),(Fiese,1958)

CHAPTER 6

Laboratory Diagnosis of Valley Fever

WHEN TRYING TO CONFIRM A CASE of valley fever, laboratory analysis may help. *Coccidioides* is a potent infecting organism, and it is important that laboratory workers take precautions when *coccidioidomycosis* is considered. Lab workers have become ill after inhaling the spores, and biosafety level 3 labs are required when working with the arthrospore-producing phase of *cocci*. Specifically, when "processing or manipulating Petri plate cultures, soil or other environmental material known to contain arthrospores, then biosafety 3 lab is required." (Biosafety and Microbiologic and biomedical laboratories)

Here are the laboratory tests for diagnosing valley fever:
- Blood test
- Sputum analysis and bronchoalveolar lavage
- Tissue biopsy
- Urinalysis
- Cerebrospinal fluid analysis
- Polymerase chain reaction (PCR)

Blood test. The most commonly used diagnostic tool is the serum laboratory test, or blood test. Serum antibodies are produced by the human immune system to fight the infection. These are known as the IgM and IgG antibodies. Patients require an intact cell mediated immunity (T-lymphocytes) to overcome this infection. The cd4 lymphocyte count, when less than 250 (normal 500-1000 cells/mm3), increases risk for *cocci* and reactivated *cocci*. (Ampel NM, Dols CL, Galgiani JN, 1993) (Ampel, 1992) (Jones J, Fleming PL, Ciesielski C, Hugh DJ, Kaplan JE, Ward JW, 1995) (Stevens, 1995)

Most patients who contract valley fever and recover will not get another cocci illness. They are immune-protected from new cases. However, immunosupression (from illness or medication) in patients may, in rare cases, cause reactivation of valley fever that had resolved.

IgM antibodies are typically detected earlier in infections, and IgG antibodies are detected later in a case of valley fever infection. Both antibodies typically drop to undetectable levels as the infection resolves. A positive blood test is reportable to the Arizona Department of Health and is considered a case of valley fever. *Coccidioidomycosis* has been reportable to the Health Department since 1997.

> *A diagnostic concern is when the serum test shows a negative IgM antibody and a positive IgG antibody. The clinician may interpret this as old infection, but it in fact may be current disease, and diagnosis is then delayed.*

When ordering routine laboratory tests for suspected valley fever, four tests are helpful: *coccidioidomycosis* serology, to see the antibodies IgM and IgG; a complete blood count (CBC); and occasionally, a sedimentation rate test and C-reactive protein test. The CBC may show either a normal or only slightly elevated white count. The white count is usually more elevated with a bacterial infection. Additionally, the eosinophils may be elevated. Eosinophilia in a CBC supports suspicion of *cocci* infection, and persistent eosinophilia is indicative of *cocci* dissemination. (Simmons, et al, Hum Pathol. 2011, 42:449-453)

Throughout the years, a variety of blood tests have been designed to detect valley fever antibodies. The most commonly used in Arizona include enzyme immune assay (EIA), and immunodiffusion. Larger laboratories in Phoenix perform a screen with the enzyme immune assay that is thought to be more sensitive but less specific for valley fever. When this is positive, an immunodiffusion is performed looking for the antibodies IgM and IgG. Typically the IgM antibody will rise in the initial week of infection, and then IgG antibodies will follow and can stay elevated for several months, later dropping to undetectable levels.

> *IgM antibodies are typically detected earlier in infections and IgG later in infection. Both antibodies typically drop to undetectable levels as the infection resolves.*
>
> *A negative blood test does not rule out valley fever. False positives also occur with valley fever.*
>
> *Sedimentation rate (ESR) and C-reactive protein (CRP) are non-specific lab tests for generalized inflammation and can be used to assess and follow response to treatment.*

When the immunodiffusion test is positive, complement fixation antibody titers can be done to give the health professional more information on the severity of the disease. Titers are a method of quantifying antibodies. The higher the level of antibodies detected in the serum, the worse the case. When the titers are greater than 1:16, the risk of dissemination is greater. Normal is less than 1:2.

Health professionals have seen critically ill patients who present with laboratory results negative for valley fever. When suspicious of valley fever, consider starting antifungal therapy before diagnostic confirmation. A negative blood test does not rule out valley fever. Repeat testing can later demonstrate a positive test. This may be a sign the immune system has recognized the fungal infection and is fighting it. Good to know, but to further confusion in the lab milieu, Kuberski, et al, demonstrated in one study that false positive IgM serology is common. Eighty-two percent of patients with IgM positive and IgG negative enzyme immunoassay (EIA) lab tests did not have *cocci* infection.

Updating blood tests are part of diagnosis as well as treatment in valley fever cases. Following titers over time helps the physician determine when treatment may be discontinued. In addition, the patient's physical signs, symptoms and medical imaging should all be part of the equation in the diagnosis and treatment process.

Demosthenes Pappagianis, M.D. is an iconic valley fever researcher and serology expert. As he stated in his paper, "Serologic Studies in Coccidioidomycosis," in 2001, "Negative serologic (as well as negative skin) tests, do not rule out *coccidioidomycosis*. And though the serologic tests have been highly successful aids, histopathology and cultural testing must be performed to complete the examination of the patient."

When a patient asks, "Do I still have the disease or not?" or "What are my titers?" I respond with more questions! I ask:

"How are your valley fever symptoms?"

"Do you still have fevers, chills or sweats?"

"Is your rash gone?"

"Do you have any headaches?"

"Are you still very tired?"

"Are you back at work full time?"

After getting these answers, I go back to the patient's latest blood test results.

A variety of factors are significant in whether a patient has a positive or negative *cocci* blood test, including immune status, timing of the blood test and confidence in the lab's reputation. In the past, not all the labs were using the same reagents or techniques, which could be related to the variance in positive tests. A recent change in lab testing kits appears to be more accurate and may reflect a decrease in false positive.

(Galgiani JN, et al) (Hedges E, Miller S., 1990) (Kuberski T, Herrig J, Pappagianis D, 2010) (Pappagianis, Application and interpretation of serologic tests, 2005, Apr. 25) (Polidge CR, et al., 2006) (Saubolle MA, McKellar PP, Sussland D, 2007) (Smith CE, Salto MT, Simons SA, 1956) (Stevens, 1995)

Most experts agree on the need for better blood testing. I will also emphasize that in this high technology medical environment, the physician's bedside diagnostic skills are very important in listening to the patient and performing a thorough exam.

Sputum or lung lavage (bronchoalveolar lavage). Here results are obtained from sputum via a productive cough or bronchoscopy for culture. The bronchoscope is wedged into the affected lung lobe when the patient is sedated. A sample is obtained by performing saline lavage for culture and analysis. This method may identify *cocci* spherules and endospores. (Sobonya R, Barbee RA, Wiens J, Trego D, 1990)

Urine analysis. Checking the urine for *cocci* is not commonly done but MiraVista Diagnostics in Indianapolis performs a *Coccidioides* quantitative antigen EIA of urine and bronchoalveolar lavage fluid. The tests are intended to help diagnose and monitor valley fever, as well as assess for possible relapse. (Mira Vista Diagnostics, Joseph Wheat, M.D.)

Tissue biopsy. If diagnosis is unclear and there is a lesion in the lung, other organ, bone, joint or skin, a needle biopsy or surgical biopsy could be performed to assess for *cocci* spherules and endospores on histopathology. This is defined as the microscopic study of diseased tissue. (Saubolle MA, McKellar PP, Sussland D, 2007)

Polymerase chain reaction. Detects the target gene for *Coccidioides* after DNA extraction from infected tissue. This test is highly specific but not widely available. (Gago S, Buitrago MJ, Clemons KV, Cuenca-Estrella M, Mirels LF, Stevens DA, 2014) (Hospenthal, 2013)

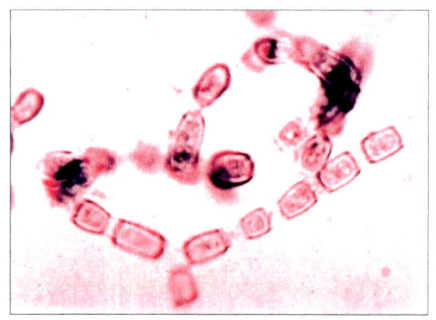

Cocci arthrospore

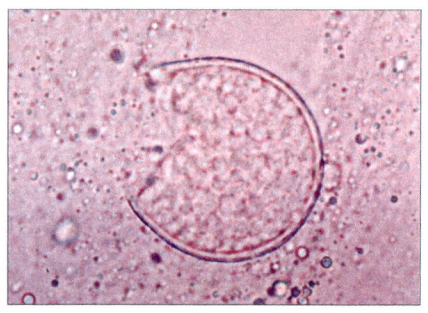

Pathological slide of rupturing spherule in lung tissue—releasing endospores.

CHAPTER 7

Valley Fever and the Lungs, Plus Some Interesting Facts

ONCE ARTHROSPORES ARE INHALED into the lung tissue, inflammation and infection cause fungal pneumonia. If an individual seeks medical attention and a chest x-ray is ordered, a spectrum of findings is possible:

- Fungal pneumonia
- Lung nodule
- Lung cavity
- Pleural effusion
- Mediastinal adenopathy (lymph node enlargement)

Fungal pneumonia. The inflammation caused by the infection clouds the lung tissue. This can affect one or more of the five lobes of the lung. Valley fever is common in the upper lobes. Multiple lung lobe involvement is more common in immunocompromised patients such as those with AIDS, or large exposures, such as people digging or working in areas with a high concentration of arthrospores, such as the outbreaks described at the end of Chapter 3. The initial

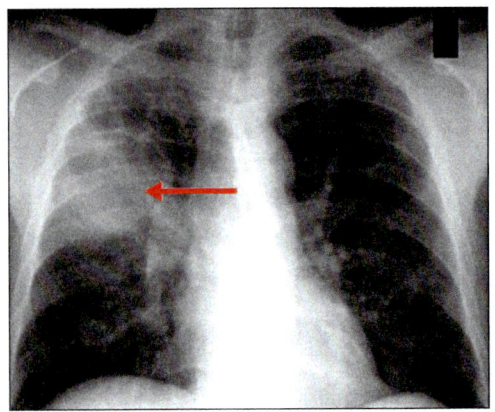

Right upper lobe cocci pnuemonia

infection of the lungs is termed primary pulmonary *coccidioidomycosis*.

Lung nodule. Lung nodules typically evolve from the original pneumonia as a residual scar and eventually become granulomas (inflammatory immune cellular residual within tissue). Granulomas can appear very similar to lung cancer. If a patient was unaware of prior *cocci* infection and is at high risk for cancer based on occupation or smoking history, a CT of the chest and lung biopsies should be considered.

The clouding of the fungal pneumonia resolves into a small nodule that completely dissipates in 90 to 95 percent of patients. Five to 10 percent of people have a permanent residual scar or a granuloma that typically causes no medical problems.

All lung nodules should be monitored for two years. In my opinion, even when a lung nodule is biopsied and determined to be *coccidioidomycosis*, the lesion should be followed whether treatment has started or not. Patients may have two or more problems at the same time, and even *cocci* lesions may enlarge, especially for high-risk patients such as diabetics, or those on immunosuppressive medication. If a lung nodule increases in

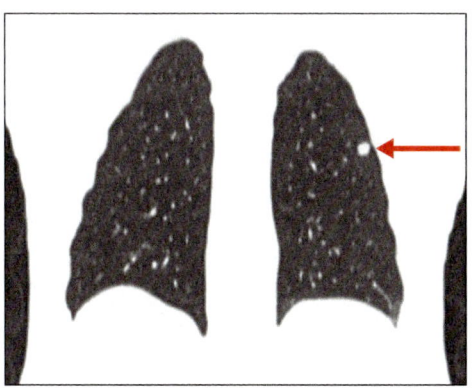

A C.T. image of LUL residual cocci nodule.

size, antifungal therapy should be considered, and with continued enlargement, surgical removal of the nodule is advised.

Lung cavities. Lung cavities occur in a nodule as the tissue breaks down. This is more common in diabetic patients. Cavities may not cause any symptoms, but bleeding may arise especially in patients on any of the growing list of anticoagulants (blood thinners) such as warfarin, Plavix, aspirin. As the cavity grows, a thoracic surgeon may require surgical removal because rupture can occur into the pleural space (space between the lung and inner chest wall). Secondary bacterial infection can

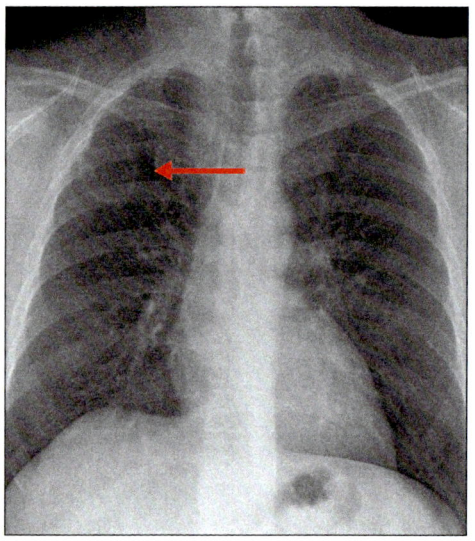

Right upper lobe cocci cavity

occur in the cavities, requiring antibiotics for treatment. (Gadkowski, B and Stout, J, Clin. Microbiol. Rev. April 2008, vol. 21, no. 2, 305-333)

Mediastinal adenopathy. Mediastinal adenopathy refers to the lymph nodes in the chest, adjacent to the heart and major blood vessels. *Cocci* pneumonia can cause these lymph nodes to enlarge and appear similar to lymphoma or lung cancer. Most of these lymph nodes will reduce in size and return to normal with resolution of the illness. If the healthcare professional is very suspicious, a mediastinal lymph node is biopsied to ensure no malignancy (such as lymphoma or lung cancer) is present. When the patient has typical valley fever signs and symptoms, consider monitoring rather than biopsy.

Pleural effusion. This happens when fluid collects outside the lung but on the inside of the chest wall (between the visceral and parietal pleura). Fluid can be withdrawn and analyzed for infection agents such as bacteria, viruses or fungi, including the spores that cause valley fever. Possible malignancy is also assessed. Increased eosinophils may also be seen in the test results in pleural effusion of *cocci* patients. (Drutz DJ, Catanzaro A, 1978) (Drutz DJ, Catanzaro A, 1978) (Freedman SI, Ang EP, Halle RS, 1986) (Galgiani JN, et al) (Galgiani, Coccidioidomycosis: A regional disease of national importance, an up-

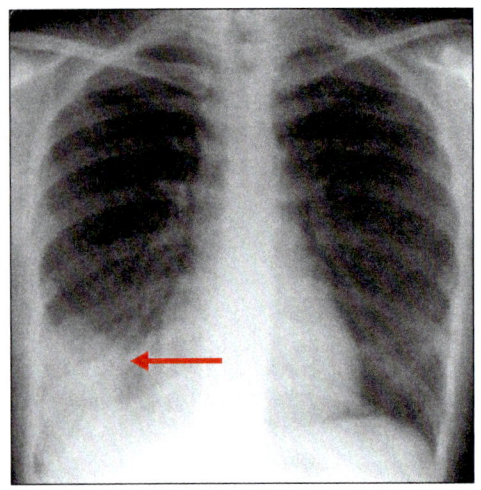

Right lower lobe pneumonia

date. Rethinking, 1999) (Hedges E, Miller S., 1990) (Hospenthal, 2013) (Hyde, 1968).

Interesting Facts
- Valley Fever can appear like cancer or tuberculosis
- Patients admitted to hospitals, especially those outside the endemic zone, are often placed in isolation until tuberculosis or another infectious disease is ruled out
- Most lung nodules and cavities resolve within one to five years

- Lung nodules and cavities need to be monitored for a total of two years to ensure resolution or residual scarring; if these lesions grow, they may need to be surgically removed
- Infections of the lung such as valley fever often look similar to cancer on radiographic imaging studies called PET scanning (positron emission test)
- PET scans should only be ordered if there is a low likelihood of cocci infection and a higher likelihood of cancer.
- PET scans may lead to unnecessary expense, biopsies and complications such as pneumothorax (lung collapse)
- Typically during an acute phase of valley fever, I order x-rays every four to eight weeks to follow the patient's evolution as the illness resolves
- Chest x-rays, and on occasion, a CT of the chest are ordered at six-month intervals to ensure stability of the lesion's size

CHAPTER 8

Valley Fever: Up Close and Personal

TO DIAGNOSE VALLEY FEVER, a thorough history and physical will be completed by the health professional followed by a determination of the extent and the severity of the disease.

According to the Arizona Department of Health Services, the reported number of valley fever sufferers in Arizona has been increasing since it became reportable in 1997. In 2011, there were 16,472 cases reported. The highest rate of infection occurred in Maricopa County followed by Pinal County and then Pima County. (2012cocci annual report): The incidence of symptomatic *cocci* in the U.S increased from 2,265 reported cases in 1998 to 22,401 in 2011. (MMWR Chap. 11 2013, 62:217-221) In Arizona, the peak season occurs from June through August and October through November. In California, late summer through fall is the peak infection period.

When a patient has a constellation of symptoms, a chest x-ray and *cocci* serology should be ordered. Other tests could also be obtained for helping clinicians determine the diagnosis—for instance, sputum gram stain culture and sensitivity, and a fungal stain and culture. The gram stain and culture and sensitivity analyses will help identify bacteria while the fungal stain will potentially show *Coccidioides* parasitic cells by microscopic examination. Antifungal therapy should be considered if the patient is clinically symptomatic. When diagnosing valley fever, the medical professional should inquire about the symptoms suggestive of the disease: headaches, joint swelling or pain, rash, fatigue, fever and cough.

Headaches are common during the primary infection, but if they persist, cerebrospinal fluid analysis in conjunction with magnetic resonance imaging (MRI), or CT of the brain can be ordered to rule out valley fever-caused meningitis. Untreated meningitis is fatal. Hydrocephalus can occur, requiring a shunt. (Galgiani JN, Cantazaro A, Cloud G, et. al., 1993) (Galgiani JN, Ampel NM, Blair J, Catanzaro A, Johnson RH, Stevens DA, Williams PL, 2005) (Galgiani JN, Canetizara A, et al, 2000) (Galgiani JN, et al) (Kirkland TN, Fierer J., 1996) (Stevens, 1995)

Joints should be examined closely and assessed for any unusual swelling or pain. The health professional should document pain or swelling of any joint in the chart.

Erythema nodosum, a rash of the lower shins, is often associated with swelling of the ankles and should be followed. Complaints of unusual back, joint or bone pain can be evaluated with bone scans, x-rays, or MRIs. The rash erythema nodosum can be treated with non-steroidal anti-inflammatory medication. Potassium iodide has been used for refractory cases of this rash.

Case Histories

Case 1

John is a 59-year-old Caucasian with no significant medical problems. He was diagnosed with right upper lobe pneumonia after seeking help for a respiratory infection. He complained of cough, fever, chills and marked fatigue.

John was given an antibiotic and cough medicine but after one week, went back to his primary care doctor. His physician was suspicious of *cocci* as his symptoms were consistent and showed minimal response to antibiotic. When questioned, John reported no unusual headaches, joint swelling, or other signs of disseminated disease but did recall a brief rash when the illness first started, which he attributed to allergy. He was placed on fluconazole, 400 mg a day, and labs were ordered for *cocci* with a follow-up chest x-ray. The valley fever anes IgG and IgM were positive and his titers were elevated. John remained on fluconazole for six months with monthly laboratory checks by his doctor, including liver enzymes and antibody testing with titers. His symptoms slowly improved and he was able to go back to work after three months but did not feel like he could perform his usual exercise routine and other hobbies until after six months of treatment. His chest radiograph was followed for three months after which time his pneumonia resolved.

After completing his treatment and medication stopped, he was instructed to call any symptoms of flare-up, especially in first few weeks.

Key Points

- Fatigue is common, so I advised him to use a graduated exercise program three to four weeks after the illness began as he could tolerate, to combat this fatigue
- John had a typical case of community-acquired pneumonia due to valley fever; clinical consideration would include starting oral antifungal medication or close observation
- The Arizona Department of Health Services recomnds all patients diagnosed with pneumonia in the mic zone be tested for valley fever

Case 2

Gail is a 75-year-old female who has medical history of atrial fibrillation, breast cancer and chronic obstructive pulmonary disease due to smoking. She developed a *cocci* lung infection. She was treated successfully and was monitored closely as the warfarin she takes for atrial fibrillation interacts with fluconazole, making her blood much thinner. Her doctor lowered her dose of warfarin by 75 percent and obtained a weekly INR for the first few weeks.

Upon completion of her treatment, although she felt much improved, she had a residual lung cavity measuring 2 x 2 cm. The cavity was followed for two years and did not change. Four years after her original diagnosis on a chest radiograph from her primary doctor, the lesion enlarged to 6 x 8 cm. A discussion ensued about the risk of the cavity, including its rupture, which could create a surgical emergency and bleeding. The options for antifungal treatment were discussed. As she had significant bleeding risk and side effects due to the antifungals (including very dry skin, marked hair loss and constipation) she consulted with a surgeon and subsequently the cavity was surgically removed. Remarkably, she was not significantly symptomatic when she had the cavity, but upon further questioning, she recalled streaks of blood on occasion in her mucous when she coughed.

Valley Fever: Up Close and Personal

Key Points

- Cavities can get secondary bacterial infections (Feldman BS and Snyder LS, 2001 Primary pulmonary coccidioidmycosis. Semin. Respir. Infect., 16:231-237)
- Cavities are more common in diabetic patients (Santelli AC, Blair JE, Roust LR, 2006. Coccidiodiomycosis in patients with diabetes mellitus. Amer. J. Med. 119:964-969.)
- Cavities can appear similar to lung cancer, especially squamous cell lung cancer (Sobonya RE, Ynez J, Klotz SA,, 2014) (Stevens, 1995)

Case 3

Gus is a 38-year-old Caucasian security guard. He was referred to the clinic for a disfiguring skin lesion on his nose. It was biopsied and shown to have *coccidioidomycosis* spherules. Gus had no recollection of being sick with pneumonia and was not immunosuppressed. Past medical history was unremarkable, and overall Gus was very healthy. He was started on 800 mg a day of fluconazole. Slowly the lesion began to heal, and the dosing was decreased over several months to 400 mg a day.

Gus was questioned about any other symptoms of extra-pulmonary disease and he reported none. He reported no bone pain or unusual headaches. After about one year of treatment, his dose was lowered to 200 mg a day and he remains on that for now. His valley fever antibodies were negative and chest x-ray is clear.

Key Points

- Patients can have disseminated disease and not ever be aware of the primary *Coccidioides* infection
- Although nasal involvement is not common, *cocci* has be seen in virtually every organ including prostate gland, eye, bones, skin, brain, etc.

Case 4

Jill is a 28-year-old African American female executive in her first trimester of pregnancy. She reports being very healthy throughout her life, but a few weeks after moving to Phoenix, she became ill and diagnosed with pneumonia.

Jill's obstetrician placed her on antibiotics, but as she was not improving, referred her to a high-risk perinatolgist who diagnosed valley fever pneumonia. Her *cocci* lab was positive and her titers were very high at 1:128, putting her in a very high-risk situation, as *cocci* in pregnancy can be fatal. A discussion on treatment fully determined she would start on intravenous Amphotercin B (or related compound) as fluconazole and other azoles have a severe teratogenic effect, particularly in the first trimester before embryogenesis has been completed. As she moved into the second trimester, the doctor discussed converting her to fluconazole, as risk was much lower after the fetus was formed. Her symptoms did improve and her titers slowly declined. Midway through her second trimester, she started on fluconazole as the IV therapy was causing renal failure and electrolyte imbalance. Jill did well and her baby was born very healthy. Her kidney function returned to normal a few weeks after delivery.

Key Points

- Fluconazole, especially in the first trimester, can cause craniofacial abnormalities and other congenital malformations
- Fluconazole has been used in second and third trimesters but it is strongly advised to have a perinatologist help make these critical decisions with documented informed consent
- African Americans and Filipinos are at higher risk of disseminated disease once they contract *cocci* infections
- Amphotercin B has been used in first trimester when clinically required
- In milder cases with low titers, observing the patient without antifungal therapy in first trimester and then introducing in second or third trimester is reasonable,

as the risk of worsening infection increases with each trimester due to the hormonal effects of pregnancy and decreased cellular immunity. (Aleck K, Bartley D, 1997) (Colivas KN, Comrie DC, 2003) (Galgiani JN, Ampel NM, Blair J, Catanzaro A, Johnson RH, Stevens DA, Williams PL, 2005) (Jick, 1999) (Zonios DI, Bennett, JE, 2008) (Stevens, 1995)

Case 5

Jay is a 55-year-old male who works at the Homeland Security office in Phoenix. He came to our office with symptoms of fever, chills, sweats, cough and recent rash on his torso described in red patches that subsided.

Jay reported there had been recent construction in and around his building, and it's been dusty especially when leaving and entering. He noticed the crew tries to clean up, but it is a mess. His lab and chest x-ray were consistent with *cocci* pneumonia and he started on antifungal therapy. After about one month, he returned to work but reported protracted fatigue.

Key Points

- Construction sites need to have dust control measures implemented and enforced
- Protected entrances and exits are advised in buildings under construction for staff protection

- Ironically, *cocci* was on the select list of agents listed in government publications that could be used in bioterrorism (until recently)

Case 6

Joe is a 29-year-old Filipino diabetic male. While walking out of a fitness center early one morning, he inadvertently walked into a plume of dust created by a landscape blower. A few days later, he came down with influenza-like symptoms: fever, chills, fatigue, sweats and headaches. He was unable work, went to urgent care and was given an antibiotic.

As his symptoms persisted and his headaches worsened, he went to his primary doctor. Given his high-risk status, he was ordered to have an MRI brain and spinal fluid analysis. The *cocci* serology was ordered and his titers were 1:64. A spinal tap was positive for meningitis. Joe was admitted to the hospital and started on intravenous antifungal with fluconazole. When he felt stable a few days later, he was discharged on 800 mg a day fluconazole by mouth. Joe was followed closely as an outpatient every three weeks initially and advised to call with any problems. His *cocci* titers slowly dropped over one year to 1:2.

Key Points

- Landscapers need to be educated about the hazards of leaf and dust blowing, especially around childcare

centers, and senior care homes. Avoid creating dust plumes in busy public areas.
- Joe is high risk for disseminate disease given that he is a Filipino male and diabetic
- Filipino and African American are at higher risk of disseminated disease once they contract *cocci* (Kirkland TN, Fierer J., 1996) (Stevens, 1995) (Malo J, Lurashchi-Monjagatta C, Wolk DM, Thompson R, Hage C, Knox K)
- *Cocci* meningitis that is NOT TREATED is 100 percent fatal
- Current recommendations are 400 mg a day for life of fluconazole
- Itraconazole can be substituted if fluconazole is not well tolerated
  - Hydrocephalus requiring shunts as well as cerebral vasculitis has been reported
- If antifungal therapy is stopped for whatever reason, recurrence is high (Galgiani J, Cantazaro A, Cloud G, et. al., 1993) (Galgiani JN, Ampel NM, Blair J, Catanzaro A, Johnson RH, Stevens DA, Williams PL, 2005) (Galgiani JN, Canetizara A, et al, 2000) (Galgiani JN, et al) (Hydrocephalus in Cocci meningitis. Case report and review of literature, 2000) (Tucker RM, Galgiani J, Denning DW, Hunson LH, et. al., 1990) (Tucker RM, Galgiani JN, Dennis DW, Hansen LH, Graybill JR, & Shark, 1999) (Nelson and Vytopil on recurrence of coccidiodal meningitis after discontinuation of Flu; JAMA Neurol 2013, 70:1586)

- Medication compliance is extremely important with valley fever meningitis (Deresinski, 1980) (Dismukes WE, Pappas PG, Sobel JD, 2003) (Drutz DJ, Catanzaro A, 1978) (Drutz DJ, Catanzaro A, 1978) (Galgiani JN, Ampel NW, Blair J2005, ISDA guidelines)

CHAPTER 9

Treatment of Valley Fever

THE INFECTIOUS DISEASES SOCIETY OF AMERICA published guidelines for health professionals treating valley fever. (Infectious Diseases 2005; 41:1217-1223) The objective was to provide recommendations to determine which patients are likely to benefit from treatment.

Mild Cases

When a patient has a mild case or minimal symptoms, no pharmacological treatment is necessarily required. Based on my own experience, I start antifungal medication when the patient appears clinically ill. For those who complain of fevers, chills, sweats and fatigue, unless medicine is contraindicated, treatment should be considered. Contraindications such as an allergy or drug interactions may make it risky to start the antifungal drug treatment. This may seem intuitive to the reader—when a patient is ill, the doctor should treat—but valley fever medication has side effects that cause concern.

Individuals suffering with valley fever will be monitored in our clinic every three to four weeks with laboratory values including *cocci* serology and titers, liver function and chest x-rays. As clinical symptoms improve, visits are spaced further out, every six to eight weeks. With improving signs and symptoms of valley fever, negative laboratory tests or titers, and resolving infiltrates on chest x-rays, medication can be decreased or discontinued. I prefer to decrease the dose of the antifungal following a decrease in valley fever symptoms rather than abruptly discontinue it. If symptoms worsen after a medication has been lowered or stopped, I will resume antifungal treatment for another month and reassess.

Severe Cases

Disseminated disease (which goes beyond the lung and creates havoc with other bodily functions) may require life-long therapy. Patients are told to call for an appointment if symptoms worsen while on or off medical therapy.

Some patients are anxious about stopping antifungal therapy, especially when they've been very ill for months or have flared up with disease while on a lower dose. I think of this as post-traumatic valley fever syndrome (not an official term, of course, but it describes what I've seen).

If medication is started on a patient with *cocci* pneumonia, and after a couple weeks the valley fever diagnosis is in question, stopping the antifungal may help in confirming clinical diagnosis (a litmus test).

I have the patient call if any symptoms reoccur or if they are concerned that they are getting worse. Some will know within a few days and may complain of fatigue, night sweats or other symptoms, and I will resume medication, then repeat lab work in two or three weeks. When necessary, I will use other diagnostic modalities to confirm diagnosis. If no issues arise, then I know that the patient either had a mild case of *cocci* or they had some other unknown and community-acquired respiratory infection.

Meningitis associated with valley fever can be fatal when fluconazole is discontinued. It is advised that fluconazole be used for the life of the patient at 400 mg a day after a diagnosis of meningitis. Itraconazole can also be considered if fluconazole is not tolerated.

Skin Test Use in Monitoring and Treatment of Valley Fever

Nielsen BioSciences developed a skin test called Spherusol® that will be available 2014 to assess cellular immune response to *Coccidioides* infections. A skin test could be used clinically to assess healthy patients to see if they've had valley fever (if they get pneumonia in the future, valley fever can be ruled out). A positive skin test is indicative of protection against *cocci*—similar to a vaccine and cannot differentiate between current or past infection. Also, a positive skin test is a good prognostic sign as it represents intact cellular immunity.

Multiple potential uses will be discussed by health professionals in the coming months as Nielsen BioScience launches Spherosol®. The FDA has approved specific indications; however it will likely be used on rheumatologic, transplant and gastroenterology patients who may be placed on immunosuppresive drugs. Obstetricians also may decide to skin test select high risk patients (see list of high risk groups in Chapter 10).

Knowing your skin test status (particularly for those soil in the endemic regions who work with such as in construction, building roads, military personnel, landscapers and farmers) would be important because if they become ill with valley fever, it could have a role in disability and workers' compensation claims.

Performing the skin test on those with acute infection may be considered, especially if known prior skin tests were negative.

Failure to develop a positive skin test in a patient with known *cocci* is a poor prognostic sign and reactivation is more common in these people.

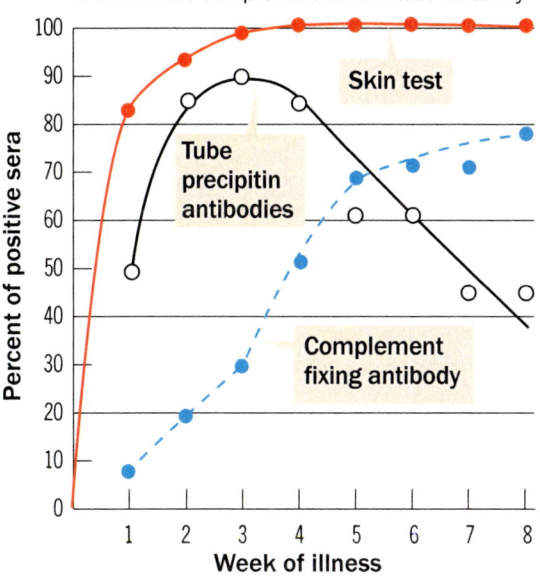

Smith, Ped Clinic N Am, 1955

Spherusol® Information

1. Spherule derived skin test antigen.
2. For intradermal injection-volar surface forearm (palm side).
3. Dosage is 0.1 milliliters.
4. Induration of 5 millimeters or greater is positive/reactive assessed at 48 hours
(Induration is a visible area of raises hardened skin).
5. Immunosuppressed patients and immunosupressive medication may inhibit response to skin test thus may not develop a positive skin test.
6. The most common adverse reaction are itching, swelling, and pain within 7 days of injection. (See prescibing information for full details.)

(Coccidioidomycosis, Drutz, Am Rev Rsp Dis, 1978) (VFACC lecture, 2010 by Elizabeth Wack, M.D., The imminent return of skin testing for Coccidioidomycosis; A primer) (Spherosol package insert prescribing information revised 2013)

Medications for Treating Valley Fever

Antifungals are drugs used for the symptomatic treatment of valley fever. There is a wide range in cost, as show below. The generic name is first; the brand name is in parentheses.

The antifungal medications known as –azoles and their cost factor:
- Ketoconazole (Nizoral) $
- Fluconazole (Diflucan) $$
- Itraconazole (Sporinox) $$$
- Voriconazole (Vfend) $$$$
- Posaconazole (Noxafil) $$$$
- Other antifungals:
  Nikkomycin-z: Unavailable—still in research
  Amphotericin and related compounds—costs vary

Nizoral (ketoconazole)
- FDA approved for valley fever
- Advised only when other effective therapy is not available
- Dosage is 200 – 400 mg per day
  Risk of liver toxicity

Also interferes with testosterone and may cause adrenal insufficiency
- Ketoconazole a imidazole, which has two nitrogen rings on molecular structure versus the three nitrogenous rings of the triazoles

Pharmacologic safety profile favors triazole oral use

Serious Side Effects
- Cardiac arrhythmia
- Anaphylaxis

Mechanism of Action
- Damages cell membrane of the fungus altering permeability.
- Assess for drug interactions especially warfarin and lipid medications such as HMG-CoA reductase inhibitors. Monitor liver function regularly.

Consider periodic cortisol and testosterone serum levels as well as a baseline EKG. An unknown cardiac problem can exist and if patient unknowingly has arrhythmia or Q-T prolongation they could be potentially be at much greater risk. Patients on multiple medications are at greater risk and pharmacist assistance is advised for drug interactions.

Diflucan (fluconazole)
- Class: triazole antifungal
- Most commonly used –azole to treat valley fever
- Can use oral or IV
- Dosage is 400 – 800 mg a day
- Doses adjust for renal failure in patients that are not on dialysis
- Pregnancy Category D
- Assess for drug interactions especially warfarin and ipid medications such as HMG-CoA reductase inhibitors. Monitor liver function regularly.

Serious Side Effects
- Can cause cardiac arrhythmia
- Steven Johnson syndrome or other dermatologic reactions

Common Side Effects
- Nausea
- Vomiting
- Headaches
- Dry skin
- Hair loss

I often suggest lip and skin moisturizers, stool softeners for constipation to mitigate side effects. Many patients use biotin and Nioxin shampoo, saying it helps prevent hair loss.

Mechanism of Action
- Inhibits fungal sterol synthesis and is considered a fungal static (does not kill the fungus but neutralizes it).

More specifically, the triazoles including fluconazole, itraconazole, voriconazole, and posoconazole inhibit essential enzyme 14-a-sterol-demethylase in the biosynthesis of ergosterol, which is key component of fungal cell membrane.

Sporonox (itraconazole)
- Class-synthetic triazole available in capsules
- Usual dose is 200 mg, two or three times a day, up to 800 mg a day
- IV form is available but reserved for severe infection
- Commonly prescribed drug for skeletal involvement of valley fever (Galgiani JN, Cantizaro A, et al. Annals of Internal Medicine, 2000. 133:676-686)
- Pregnancy Category C
- Can cause cardiac arrhythmia, electrolyte imbalance and congestive heart failure
- Requires gastric acid for absorption, so it is best to take capsules with meals
- Absorption is improved with cola drinks or cranberry juice (Jaruratanasirikul S, Kleepkaew A,

Influence of acidic beverage (Coca-Cola) on absorption of itraconazole. Eur. J Clinic Pharmacol. 1997:52-73) (Lange D, Pavao JH, Wu J, et al. Effects of cola beverage on the bioavailability of itraconazole in the presence of H2 blocker. J Clin Pharmacol 1997; 37:535)
- Assess for drug interactions, especially warfarin

Side Effects/Drug considerations
- Monitor liver enzymes and serum itraconazole levels. Stop HMG-CoA reductase inhibitors if possible. Consider baseline EKG to assess heart rhythm.

Patients often prefer itraconazole to fluconazole. It causes less hair loss although is more expensive.

If patients are on antacid medication or proton pump inhibitors such as Protonix, Prevacid, or H2 blockers such as Zantac, it is advised that they take these at a different time of day than when they take itraconazole as it could potentially affect absorption of medication.

Vfend (voriconazole)
- Class A triazole antifungal
- Dose 200 – 400 mg a day
  Take one hour before or after meals; oral viability independent of gastric acid and high fat meals may decrease absorption

- Consider monitoring blood levels as a 50 percent increase in dose increases serum level by 150 percent (Hope WW, Population pharmakinetics of triazole antfungal agent and voriconazole in adults. Antimicro Agent S Chemo Ther 2012. 56:526)

Mechanism of Action
- Inhibits fungal sterol synthesis.
- Assess for drug interactions especially warfarin, lipid medications and proton pump inhibitors.

Melanoma and squamous cell cancer of the skin has been seen with voriconazole as well as photosensitivity (optic neuritis and optic disc edema).

Typically used for failure of other medications to work effectively. (Micrometics) (Miller DD, Cowen EW, Nguyen JC, et. al., 2010) (Zonios DI, Bennett, JE, 2008) (Morice C, Archer A, Soufir N, Michel M, Comoz F, Leroy D, Verneuil L, 2010)

Noxafil (posaconazole)
- Class – triazole
- Dosage 200 –800mg a day; usually 400 mg twice a day
- Oral suspension 100 mg delayed release tablet approved 11/2013
- Requires fatty meal for absorption
- Very expensive

Mechanism of Action
- Blocks synthesis of key components of cell membrane.
- Monitor liver enzymes and for drug interactions.
- Consider baseline EKG because arrhythmias can occur.
- Typically used for cases resistant to other medications.

Nikkomycin-z is currently not available. Future studies are planned.
Mechanism of Action
- This drug inhibits chitin synthase activity and chitin incorporation into the spherule and endospore cell wall.

Amphotericin B deoxycholate
- Amphotericin B is a polyene antifungal agent used for severe cases as well as valley fever during pregnancy
- New lipid formulations are thought to be safer
- Amphotericin B and other lipid formulations can cause electrolyte imbalances, cardiac arrhythmia, low blood pressure, fever, chills and renal failure
- Pregnancy Category B

- Dose – 0.5 to 1.5 mg/kg per day (Amphotericin B lipid complex in the treatment of invasive fungal infections, 2005. Zonios DI, Bennett JE. 2008)

Mechanism of action
- Binds sterols in fungal cell wall creating disruption, and damage to cellular membrane.

Here is a list of some drugs that will increase concentration in the blood and potentially become dangerous when –azole antifungal therapy is used:

- Warfarin
- Statins
- Benzodiazepines
- Calcium channel blockers
- Alprazolam
- Cyclosporine
- Cephalosporin
- Fexofenadine
- Zolpidem
- Methadone

Drugs and substances that decrease –azole concentration in the blood, thus becoming less effective when administered:
- Antacids
- Carbamzepine

- Grapefruit juice
- H2 inhibitors
- Phenytoin
- Proton pump inhibitors
- St. John's Wort

These lists are not complete, and multiple medication interactions are known. Ask your physician and pharmacist before taking antifungal along with your usual medications. (Micrometics) (Physicians Desk Reference) (Zonios DI, Bennett, JE, 2008) (Tiphine M, Letscher-Bru V, Herbrecht R, 1999)

CHAPTER 10

Risk Groups

THE FOLLOWING IS A LIST OF PATIENTS at higher risk for a severe case once infected with the *Coccidioides* arthrospores:

- HIV/AIDS—greater risk when CD4 lymphocyte counts are under 250
- Age greater than 60 years old
- Cancer patients, lymphoma patients, those undergoing chemotherapy
- Organ transplant patients on anti-rejection drugs
- Infants with evolving immunity
- Immunosuppressive medication
- Race, including African-American, Filipino and Asian
- Males show a higher infection rate that is possibly occupation related
- Pregnant women
- Immune status, if weakened

(Ampel NM, Dols CL, Galgiani JN, 1993) (Ampel, 1992) (Blair JE, Mayer AP, Currier J, Files JA, Nu Q, 2008) (Peterson LR,

Marshall SL, Barton-Dixon C, Hajjeh RA, Lindsey MD, Warnock DW, et al., 2004) (Dismukes WE, Pappas PG, Sobel JD, 2003) (Drutz DJ, Catanzaro A, 1978) (Drutz DJ, Catanzaro A, 1978) (Galgiani JN, et al) (Galgiani, Coccidioidomycosis: A regional disease of national importance, an update. Rethinking, 1999) (Huang JY, Bristow B, Shafir S, Sorvillo F, 2012) (Kirkland TN, Fierer J., 1996) (Leake JA, Mosley DG, England B, et. al, 2000) (Rosenstein NE, Emery KW, Werner SB, et al., 2001)

People in high-risk groups are more likely to have a protracted course of valley fever and its disseminated disease (outside the lungs). The infection normally stimulates T-lymphocytes, which are essential for protective immune response and controlling the infection.

It is common when a patient recovers from valley fever that they are immune and protected from a recurrence. Rarely, reactivation of prior *Coccidioides* infection may occur. This would typically be in an immunosuppressed patient, such as in one with HIV or an individual getting immunosuppressive medication such as a transplant patient or an individual on tumor necrosis factor (TNF) blocker medications, possibly for rheumatologic disorders or gastrointestinal disorders.

Tumor necrosis factor is a small protein cytokine involved in cell communication acting through cell receptors. It is involved with regulation of immunity.

Disregulation can lead to a variety of diseases, thus TNF blockers can improve these illnesses at the risk of immunosuppression.　(Cytokine, inflammation and pain. Jun Ming Zhang. **www.ncbi.nlm.nih.gov**)

Here are five tumor necrosis factor blockers:
- Remicade (infliximab)
- Enbrel (etanercept)
- Humira (adalimumab)
- Cimzial (certolizumab)
- Simponi (golimumab)

　(Anti-TNF-Drugs. (n.d.). American College of Rheumatology) (Retrieved from **www.rheumatology.org**)

Here is an analysis of the risk factor groups:
HIV/AIDS – Infectious disease with HIV and AIDS correlates with CD4 lymphocyte count. The lower the count,(especially below 250cells/mm3) the higher the risk of infection with *cocci*. Ten percent of HIV patients in the endemic regions get valley fever each year. (Ampel NM, Dols CL, Glagiani JN, 1993. Coccidioidomycosis in the HIV-infected patient, diagnosis and treatment. AIDS Reader, 12-15)

Age – Increased incidence and severity is seen in elderly patients. (Blair JE, Mayer AP, Currier J, et al. 2008. Coccidioidomycosis in elderly persons. Clinical infectious diseases, 47 (12), 1513-1518)

Race – Filipino and African Americans have higher risk of disseminated disease.

Cancer – Immunosuppression from cancer and effects of treatment.

Pregnancy – Risk of disseminated disease increases with each trimester. It is felt that the decreased cellular immunity in pregnancy and the hormones of pregnancy including estradiol and progesterone nourish the growth of the fungus. (Drutz DJ, Huppert M, Sun SH, et al. 1981. Human sex hormones stimulate growth and maturation of cocci immitis. Infect Immun. 32:897-907)

Upon examination of the valley fever patient, risk stratification and assessment for extra-pulmonary disease is very important. Upon each follow-up visit, continue to ask questions that could be suggestive of disseminated disease including headaches, blurred vision and focal bone pain or joint pain/swelling.

For further reference regarding the epidemiology of valley fever, see the chapter titled, "Expanding Understanding of Epidemiology Of Coccidioidomycosis in the Western Hemisphere," by Rafael Laniado-Laborin. *Coccidioidomycosis: Sixth International Symposium*, Ed. Clemons, Karl V., Laniado-Laborin, Rafael, Stevens, David A. Annals of the New York Academy of Sciences, Volume 1111, pages 19-34.

CHAPTER 11

Case Rates and Epidemiology

VALLEY FEVER IS A REPORTABLE DISEASE to the Department of Health Services in Arizona. Valley fever causes a significant amount of community acquired pneumonia, and one study showed 29 percent of community-acquired pneumonia is due to cocci. (Valdivia L, Nix D, Wright M, et al. 2006, June. Coccidioidomycosis as a common cause of community-acquired pneumonia. Emerging Infectious Disease Journal, 12 (8))

When a person arrives at urgent care or their physician's office with symptoms of severe bronchitis or pneumonia, valley fever should be considered and cocci serology should be ordered. The Arizona Department of Health Services recommends that anybody with community-acquired pneumonia in the endemic zone should be tested for valley fever.

Case Rates

Valley fever is endemic in southwestern United States, including Arizona, California, Southwest New Mexico, Nevada and West Texas. Parts of Centr and Mexico are also endemic regions. The United States has an estimated 150,000 – 200,000 cases per year. There have been increasing case reports after significant dust storms (haboobs), rainy season after periods of droughts, and earthquakes with associated mud slides. (Increase in reported coccidioidomycosis – United States 1998-2011, 2013) (Kolivras K, Comrie KN, 2003) (Sunenshine RH, Anderson, Erhort L, et al., 2007) (Talamantes J, Behseta S, Zender CS, 2007) (Tamerius JD, Comrie DC, 2011),(Arizona Department of Health Services)

Percent positive skin test

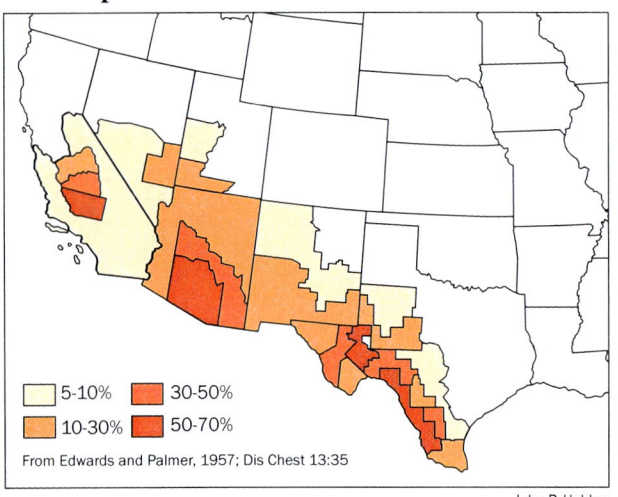

From Edwards and Palmer, 1957; Dis Chest 13:35

John P. Holden

Valley fever cases by Arizona county, 2012

	Cases	Cases per 100,000 population	Average cases per 100,000 pop. (2007-2011)
Apache	17	23.5	17.7
Cochise	48	36.7	30.8
Coconino	48	35.7	21.0
Gila	49	91.4	57.2
Graham	33	88.4	57.4
Greenlee	2	23.3	16.4
La Paz	25	119.6	108.4
Maricopa	10.116	260.4	195.8
Mohave	109	53.7	43.7
Navajo	39	36.1	26.0
Pima	1,555	157.0	122.9
Pinal	774	98.9	136.8
Santa Cruz	19	39.0	25.7
Yavapai	53	25.0	18.1
Yuma	33	16.1	8.3
Arizona	**12,920**	**198.8**	**149.0**

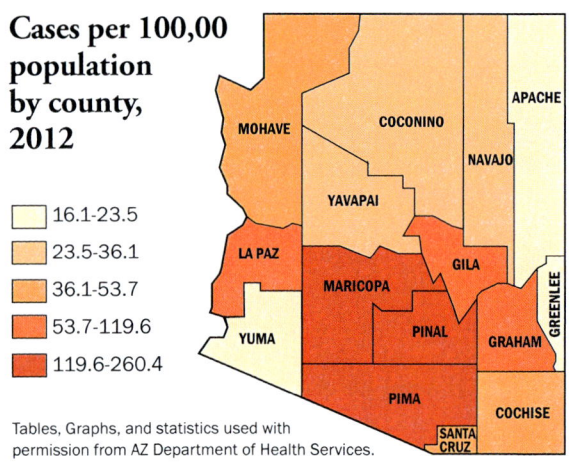

Cases per 100,00 population by county, 2012

- 16.1-23.5
- 23.5-36.1
- 36.1-53.7
- 53.7-119.6
- 119.6-260.4

Tables, Graphs, and statistics used with permission from AZ Department of Health Services.

Valley fever case reports in Arizona 1994–2013

1994 – 578	2001 – 2,301	2008 – 4,768
1995 – 623	2002 – 3,118	2009 – 10,233
1996 – 655	2003 – 2,695	2010 – 11,883
1997*– 958	2004 – 3,667	2011 – 16,467
1998 – 1,474	2005 – 3,518	2012 – 12,920
1999 – 1,812	2006 – 5,535	2013 – 7,113
2000 – 1,917	2007 – 4,832	2014 – 3,505†

*In 1997, valley fever became reportable to the Arizona Department of Health Services.
†Figure is for January - June 2014

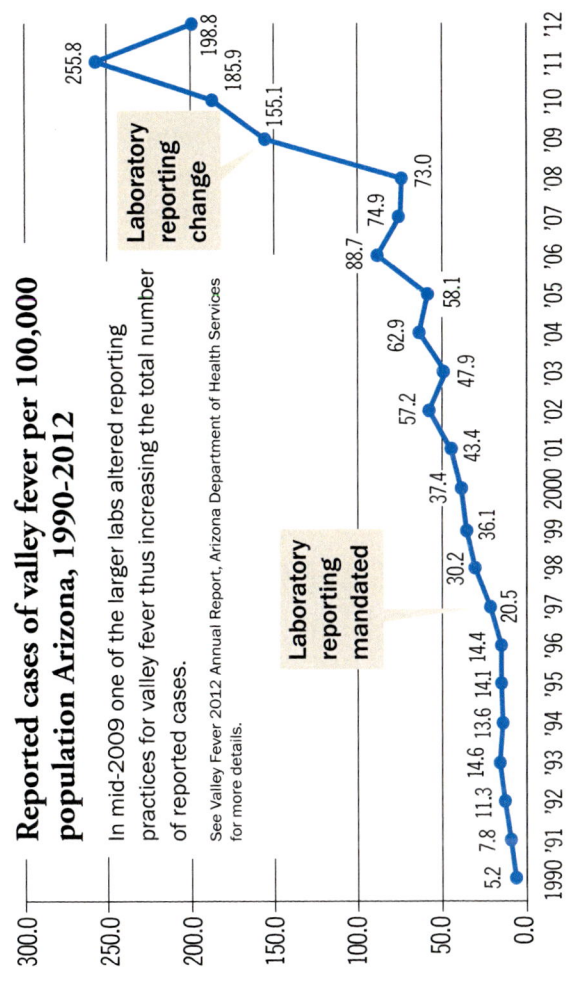

Reported cases and rates by age groups, 2012

Age Group* (years)	Cases	Cases per 100,000
<5	59	13.3
5-14	499	54.6
15-24	1387	150.6
25-34	1,857	214.5
35-44	2,215	267.3
45-54	2,175	260.00
55-64	1,923	257.0
65-74	1,587	294.6
75-84	866	295.2
85+	299	275.7

*Age could not be ascertained for 53 cases (approximately 0.4% of all cases)

Environmental triggers for increased valley fever illness reports:

- Interestingly, after a significant dust storm in 1977, spores blew from the Bakersfield area to San Francisco, where an epidemic was noted
- After the Ventura county earthquake in 1994, increased case rates were seen as mudslides created dust plumes, as well as disturbed soil releasing spores (Schneider E, Hajjeh R, Spiegel R, Jibson R, Harp E, Marshall G, et al., 1997)

- Dust storms (haboobs) and Monsoon weather place residents at risk for inhaling the cocci spores.

Case rates are also thought to increase in association with increased precipitation that was preceded by a drought. Cycles of drought and precipitation have been linked with case rate increases. Experts refer to this as the "grow and blow" theory.

Grow and Blow Theory

During periods of significant drought, arthrospores lie dormant in the soil. Being a hardy, virulent organism,

California cocci case rates 1998-2013

Year	Cases	Year	Cases
1998	719	2005	2,885
1999	939	2006	3,131
2000	840	2007	2,991
2001	1,538	2008	2,597
2002	1,727	2009	2,488
2003	2,091	2010	4,622
2004	2,641	2011	5,627
2005	2,885	2012	4,431
2006	3,131	2013	3,272
2007	2,991		

Source: The Center of Disease Control and Prevention

fewer competitors exist in the soil. When significant rains follow such dormancy during the winter season, spores germinate. When the heat of the summer dries out the soil and the dust storms ensue, large quantities of arthrospores become airborne and can infect populations of humans and animals. (Colivas KN, Comrie DC, 2003) (Comrie, 2005) (Saubolle MA, McKellar PP, Sussland D, 2007) (Smith CE, Beard RR, 1946a) (Smith CE, Beard RR, Rosenberger HG, Whiting EG, 1946) (Tamerius JD, Comrie DC, 2011)

Commonalities of the Endemic Zones

Valley fever case rates are more common in the Southwestern United States. This region is often referred to as the lower Sonoran life zone, which has vegetation common with the deserts of the southwest United States and Mexico. These deserts include the Sonoran, Mohave and Chihuahuan. Here are their common characteristics:

- Low altitude
- Warm winters
- Hot summers
- Alkaline sandy soil
- Arid climate
- Minimal rainfall—five to 20 inches per year

(Galgiani JN, et al) (Galgiani, Coccidioidomycosis: A regional disease of national importance, an update. Rethinking, 1999) (Increase in reported coccidioidomycosis – United States 1998-2011, 2013) (Laniado-Laborin, 2007) (Kirkland TN, Fierer J., 1996) (Talamantes J, Behseta S, Zender CS, 2007)

Valley fever is reported in Arizona, California, New Mexico and Nevada, but not in Texas. It is difficult to track the extent of infection in other states and countries since it is not reportable there. Valley fever is a reportable disease to health departments in the following states, according to Centers for Disease Control:

States that report valley fever to health departments

- Arizona
- California
- Delaware
- Louisiana
- Maryland
- Michigan
- Minnesota
- Missouri
- Montana
- Nebraska
- Nevada
- New Hampshire
- New Mexico
- North Dakota
- Ohio
- Rhode Island
- Utah
- Washington
- Wyoming

Some experts feel that due to the significant dust storms and monsoons propelling spores high into the atmosphere as well as climate change, *cocci* will increase in non-endemic regions. The Phoenix haboob of 2011 was estimated to be over 5,000 feet high and 100 miles wide.

The National Oceanic and Atmospheric Administration satellite imagery has demonstrated dust from the Sahara Desert in Africa reaching South America and then Florida. Hence, it is possible that *cocci* rains down throughout the United States after Arizona's dust storms. Arizona gets several of these dust storms every summer and monsoon rains often follow them.

An increase in *coccidioidomycosis* has been identified in animal dens in endemic areas presumably due to increase moisture and nitrogenous waste. Construction projects (digging foundations for housing developments), living near open desert, experiencing windy conditions while hiking and other outdoor activities can create unique hazards to local communities in endemic areas.

CHAPTER 12

Clinical Perspectives

THIS CHAPTER IS A REVIEW of most of the information in this book. It is provided as a reference to doctors and patients alike with the hope that it will underscore the attention that must be given to a possible case of valley fever.

Valley fever can present as similar to other respiratory infections, and it is important to consider its presence with any severe bronchitis, pneumonia, lung lesion or lung cavity seen in patients who live in or who have visited Arizona and other places where the disease is most prevalent. Travel history is important—health professionals can determine regional diseases their patients may have been exposed to while away from home.

Assessing the patient's history, a physical exam, finding serum antibodies and a review of chest x-rays are required for diagnosing valley fever. Stratifying a person's risk of extra-pulmonary disease is important, keeping in mind their health history (i.e., diabetes, cancer, immunosuppressive medication and immunosuppressive illnesses) as well as race and pregnancy status.

When the diagnosis is confirmed and patients are

being treated, they will typically follow up in the clinic every three to four weeks in the first couple months. A review of symptoms, lab work including *cocci* serology and titers, as well as liver function tests assessing for drug toxicity, are all performed. Even when patients with mild cases are not placed on antifungal therapy, they are asked to follow up and call if signs and symptoms begin.

Serum can be sent to laboratories familiar with valley fever testing. For example, the University of California at Davis does these tests and appropriate forms can be found on their website with associated costs. Also, larger regional hospitals often perform *cocci* lab testing or will send serum to affiliated labs.

As patients who are being treated clinically improve, such as when lab tests and a chest radiograph demonstrate a resolving infection, antifungal therapy is gradually lowered, then stopped. Patients are told to call if symptoms flare up after medication is lowered or stopped. On occasion, patients can be highly anxious about stopping therapy especially if they were significantly impacted by the illness. When clinical signs and symptoms flare after cessation, I typically give another month of an –azole therapy and then reassess.

If many months go by without resolution of the illness, then it must be determined if *cocci* is the issue or if another problem is occurring. On occasion, when individuals just don't seem be fully recovering and their symptoms appear to have evolved into a more chronic case, I advise taking yet another thorough history and having another physical by their physician or health professional.

For the enduring fatigue common in valley fever patients, a graduated exercise program and physical therapy may help by igniting endorphins and cytokines that help the person have more energy.

CHAPTER 13

Prevention of Valley Fever

PREVENTING VALLEY FEVER is difficult as the arthrospores blow easily through the air. Even in highly endemic zones, it is hard to know where the greater concentration of arthrospores exists. Preventative measures include:

- Keeping construction sites wet to minimize dust
- Consider wearing an N-95 mask if working with soil (this should help minimize risk of direct exposure) and make sure your mask is NIOSH tested and approved
- A mask can benefit particularly when planting bushes, doing irrigation work, shoveling, gardening, sweeping dusty garages, driveways and patios
- Plant grass and include paving in home landscaping
- Minimize use of blowers; safety rules need to be discussed with landscape workers who use these blowers around senior centers, day care centers, schools, etc.

Valley Fever is the 'Orphan Disease'

One has to ask that if valley fever is such a health concern in the Southwest then why is there not more being done to find a medical cure and a vaccine? If better treatment was available, billions of dollars would be saved and a significant reduction in the health care costs of Arizona and California citizens would be possible.

Valley fever is a rare disease, and it is thought that fewer than 200,000 are infected each year in the U.S. Rare diseases are labeled "orphan diseases." According to the National Institutes of Health (NIH) website, more than 6,800 rare diseases affect over 25 to 30 million people. The big picture illuminates why there have been delays in finding better treatment for valley fever. This may also be confounded by the fact that in the past, *cocci* was brushed off by many as a mild disease and the misperception by many lay people that if you live in the endemic area you probably have had it and didn't know it.

The rare disease provides less incentive for companies to search for cures because returns on their investment would be small compared to the many other diseases that need research and investment. This unfortunate fact was recognized when Congress passed the Orphan Drug Act in 1983, which provides incentives for drug companies to develop treatment for rare diseases.

The National Institute of Health (NIH) says it invested $3.5 billion toward rare diseases in 2011, and $750 million went toward orphan disease research projects.

Research grants have been allocated to *cocci* from the FDA's Office of Orphan Product Development, and to NIH, as well as to private groups and grassroots efforts, through University of Arizona.

All financial help is welcome, despite the tremendous costs of developing drugs, pharmaceutical trials, FDA approval and manufacturing of treatments such as Nikkomycin-z and a future vaccine.

CHAPTER 14

Valley Fever in Dogs

DOGS ARE PARTICULARLY SUSCEPTIBLE to valley fever in Arizona and California endemic counties. I am not a veterinarian, but I am often asked about dogs with valley fever. Patients have asked if they could have contracted the disease from their dogs. The answer is no.

Similar to humans, dogs have to first inhale the arthrospores to become ill. Valley fever is not contagious between humans or between animals and humans.

Symptoms of valley fever in dogs include:
- Cough
- Lethargy
- Decreased appetite
- Weight loss
- Shortness of breath
- Fever
- Lameness
- Skin lesions

As in humans, the infection can spread to the nervous system causing seizures as well as bone and joint involvement. Lymph glands and swollen joints are possible. Thus if your dog is ill, your veterinarian can order the laboratory test for valley fever and if required start antifungal treatment—usually fluconazole, as in humans.

The drug studies conducted by veterinarian Lisa Shubitz, DVM at the University of Arizona with Nikkomycin-z are promising: however more drugs needs to be developed. The science is there for improved medical treatments and vaccines, but the financial backing is not.

Other animals have contracted valley fever including cats (less frequently than dogs), cattle, horses and llamas; zoo animals including tigers, bears and apes. Occasionally dolphins and otters contract valley fever from arthrospores that have blown out to sea.

CHAPTER 15

The Economic Impact of Valley Fever

THE ECONOMIC IMPACT OF *COCCI* is quite significant. Consider not only the cost of hospital, urgent care and medical office visits but also the loss of productivity from inability to work for both short and long-term disability.

Cocci has been a financial strain on the military since World War II. Many bases and an estimated 350,000 active military personnel are in endemic zones, and soldiers for decades have been getting *cocci*. Prisons, especially in California, are seeing high rates of valley fever at a significant cost burden to taxpayers, as hospitalizations are required.

The California Department of Public Health reported from 2000-2011, there were 25,217 *coccidioidmycosis* hospitalizations costing more than $2 billion in hospital charges. (California department of public health. Coccidioidomycosis yearly summary report 2001 – 2010)

A study by the Arizona Department of Health Services in 2007 demonstrated that 1,735 *cocci* related hospital discharges at a cost of $86 million averaged $50,000 per hospital stay. Multiply this year over year with inflation

Cost

Total charges associated with valley fever hospitalizations in non federal facilities in Arizona 2003-2013

	Total (2012 dollars)	
	Primary	Primary or Secondary
2003	$35,841,244	$56,077,190
2004	$44,356,120	$68,142,341
2005	$47,775,374	$67,684,950
2006	$76,173,631	$108,673,079
2007	$63,368,983	$93,172,625
2008	$64,947,432	$90,337,944
2009	$81,650,772	$111,962,812
2010	$78,916,128	$112,143,360
2011	$75,015,531	$112,578,548
2012	$68,627,476	$102,686,897
Total	**$636,672,691**	**$923,459,746**

and the cost is billions of dollars. Also, 75 percent of patients missed work for one month (median 14 days). One in four patients saw their doctor at least 10 times in the medical clinics. (Arizona Department of Health Services) (Tsang CA. Anderson SM. Imholte SB. Erhart LM. Et al, Enhanced surveillance of Coccidioidomycosis, Arizona, USA. 2007-2008. Emerging Infectious Diseases. 2010:16(11): 1738-44.

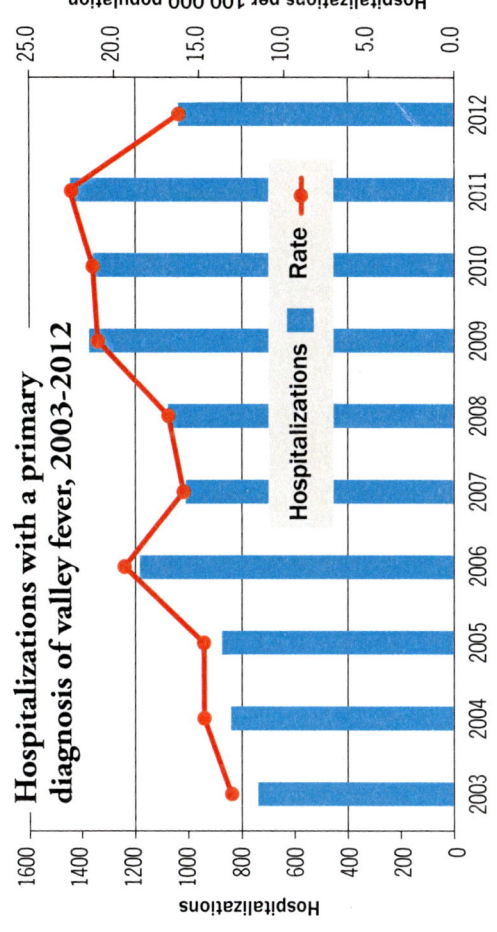

Deaths attributable to valley fever by county 2012

	Primary cause of death	Primary or secondary cause of death
Apache	0	0
Cochise	1	1
Coconino	0	0
Gila	1	1
Graham	0	0
Greenlee	0	0
La Paz	0	0
Maricopa	13	21
Mohave	0	0
Navajo	0	0
Pima	7	11
Pinal	3	5
Santa Cruz	0	0
Yavapai	0	0
Yuma	0	0
Arizona	**25**	**39**

In 2012 there were 1070 hospitalizations for patients with valley fever as the primary diagnosis at a cost of $103 million. (Arizona Department of Health Services

2012 Valley fever annual report). This is up significantly from $56 million in 2003.

Coccidioidomycosis-associated Deaths

The valley fever death rate may be underreported because if someone dies of pneumonia and a cause of infection is not identified, it cannot be appropriately counted. In the *Journal of Emerging Infectious Diseases* it was reported that between 1990 and 2008 there were 3,089 *coccidioidomycosis*-associated deaths among U.S. residents. Those at highest risk were men, people over 65, Hispanics, Native Americans and residents of California or Arizona. (Huang JY, Bristow B, Shafir S, Sorvillo F, 2012)

Men have more occupational risk, possibly accounting for their higher mortality. Deaths due to valley fever were reported in all states, which can be attributed to mobility in our society.

According to the *Milwaukee Journal,* Steve Ueker, the 52-year-old son of Milwaukee Brewers broadcaster Bob Uecker, died in a Milwaukee hospital of San Joaquin Valley fever in 2012. Wisconsin is clearly a non-endemic state.

I am sad to report that one of our clinic patients who worked as a mechanic and was diagnosed with primary pulmonary *cocci* died not from the disease directly but a protracted dermatologic reaction, Steven Johnson syndrome, caused by his antifungal medication.

Vaccine Development

Antigens from the fungal spherule cell wall have been isolated in an effort stimulate a protective immune response that will allow safe and effective vaccine to be developed. Also important are adjuvants that can enhance the immune response to vaccines. The immunology is complex and beyond the scope of this book.

Unfortunately, funding has markedly decreased and only a select few universities are working on this. Dr. Garry Cole and Dr. Chiung-Yu Hung's group at the University of Texas San Antonio, Dr. Galgiani and researchers at University of Arizona have been major contributors to the science of developing a *cocci* vaccine. In California, the Valley Fever Americas Foundation and the Valley Fever Vaccine Project (VFVP) of America have also put effort into funding vaccine. Earlier attempts to develop a defined vaccine against *cocci* have failed. (Cole GT, Sun SH, 1985) (Cox RA, Magee DM, 2004) (Fierer J, Waters C, Walls L, 2006) (Herr RA, Hung CY, Cole GT, 2007)

However, recent results using a live vaccine have been encouraging. **In fact, this live vaccine has been found to be 100 percent effective in pre-clinical studies.** (Xue, J., C.-Y. Hung, D. Selby, and G.T. Cole. 2009. A genetically-engineered live attenuated vaccine of Coccidioides protects BALB/c mice against coccidioidomycosis. Infect. Immun. 77: 3196-3208)

CHAPTER 16

Fast Fascinating Facts and Resources

- Valley Fever is caused by the fungus coccidioidomycosis and two species are known, Coccidioides immitis and Coccidioides posadasii
- *Coccidioidomycosis* is a respiratory disease caused by a soil fungus
- Other names for *coccidioidomycosis* include valley fever, desert fever, San Joaquin Valley fever and *cocci*
- Originally, many people referred to valley fever as Wernicke-Posadasii disease
- An arthrospore is a barrel-shaped spore in the soil existing in a mycelium
- Arthrospores measure 3 to 5 microns
- Spherules can grow to more than 75 microns in diameter and release their content of endospores by rupturing
- Once an arthrospore is inhaled, it changes form in about 72 hours from a barrel-shaped cell arthrospore to a spherule
- Spherules, once they rupture, release endospores

- The term valley fever originated in the San Joaquin Valley where the link was originally made between the fungus and the illness by Ernest C. Dickson, M.D.
- Valley fever illness can present very similar to any other community-acquired pneumonia
- When a health professional suspects valley fever, *cocci* serology is advised according to the Arizona Department of Health
- Valley fever has been a reportable disease since 1997 and case rates have soared
- Valley fever is a common cause of pneumonia in Arizona
- Valley fever is the second most common reported disease to the Arizona Department of Health
- Utilization of a new EIA blood test kit 2014 for cocci appears more accurate and case rates have declined (less false positives -hence reduced case rate)
- Disseminated (extra-pulmonary disease) can spread to bone, skin and meninges, essentially any organ
- Arthritis pain (arthralgias) can occur especially in ankle and knee joints as result of *cocci* infection
- The valley fever fungus has been identified in the prostate and eye
- Valley fever meningitis is a serious extra-pulmonary illness requiring life-long therapy

- Fluconazole, 400 mg a day for life, is advised for *cocci* meningitis
- High-risk patients for valley fever include those with HIV, diabetes, cancer, those who are undergoing chemotherapy, lymphoma, pregnancy, infants, males, African-Americans and Filipinos
- Skin testing studies demonstrated 60 percent of patients who contract valley fever have no symptoms or minimal symptoms, and 40 percent of those become symptomatic
- It is estimated that 0.5 to 1 percent of those who test positive for valley fever may have extra-pulmonary disease
- Dr. Charles Smith, M.D. is credited for defining much of the epidemiology of valley fever by working with skin testing
- Dr. Charles Smith was a colleague at Stanford with Dr. Dickson
- Three percent of people in the endemic region contracted valley fever as evidenced by positive per skin tests every year
- These skin tests have not been available in the U.S. for over 20 years until 2014 with Nielsen BioScience release of Spherusol®
- In 1900, Dr. W. Ophuls identified *coccidioidomycosis* to be a fungus and not a protozoan

- The blood test for valley fever can be a false negative or false positive
- A negative test does not rule out valley fever—clinical acumen and correlation are required for an accurate diagnosis
- Immunosuppressive medication such as prednisone, transplant anti-rejection drugs, anti-TNF can predispose for a worse case of valley fever
- The first known case of valley fever was seen in a man named Domingo Ezcurra in 1893
- Alejandro Posadas and Robert Wernicke treated Domingo Ezcurra in an Argentinean hospital
- Alejandro Posadas, a young medical student at that time, has been recognized for his initial work with Domingo Ezcurra, and the species *Coccidioidomycosis posadasii* is named in his honor as well as the medication posaconazole
- Common signs and symptoms of valley fever include, chills, night sweats and fatigue
- Fatigue seems to be the most prevalent symptom of valley fever
- Most rashes are thought to be hypersensitivity reactions and include erythema nodosum, erythema multiforme, which can occur with valley fever
- Valley fever is contracted when inhaling arthrospores that have been blown into the air from the soil. It also

has been inhaled from fomites (objects capable of carrying transmission of an infectious agent) such as mechanics working on cars or plants such as cacti sent to other states
- Natural disasters such as dust storms, earthquakes, mudslides, haboobs and monsoons have all been associated with increased cases of *coccidioidomycosis*
- It is very important to monitor liver enzymes and watch for drug interactions in patients on antifungal therapy as these medications can cause liver injury as well as increased effectiveness levels of many other drugs
- Athletes such as Gary Craft, a PGA golfer, and Conner Jackson, a former Arizona Diamondbacks baseball player, contracted valley fever while competing in Arizona, and the disease had a significant effect on their careers
- Filipino and African-Americans are much more likely to have disseminated *cocci* infection to other organs if they become infected with valley fever
- Dry alkaline soil, warm winters, minimal rainfall and low altitude are common in the endemic zones of valley fever
- It may be necessary to perform either bronchoscopy to obtain secretions or to do a needle biopsy to obtain tissue for diagnosis of valley fever

- Life zones refer to an area of geography, which is characterized by climate, and a dominant set of plants and animals
- Valley fever is endemic in the lower life zones—the desert conditions
- Pregnant valley fever patients should be followed closely by their health professionals, as well as by a perinatologist
- The first identified Arizona *cocci* case was in 1937
- Until recently, *cocci* was on the government's list of select agents that can be used in bioterrorism due its virulent nature
- The bioterrorism aspect of valley fever may also be responsible for the fact that there is no cure yet
- Fossil evidence suggests *cocci* has been infecting humans and animals over the last 8,500 years (Mycologia September/October 2006 vol. 98 no. 5 669-677)

RESOURCES
For patients and health care professionals:

- **John Galgiani, M.D.,** Valley Fever Center for Excellence, University of Arizona (**www.vfce.arizona.edu/**) provides comprehensive information and resources for the public and physicians

- **Valley Fever Alliance of Arizona Clinicians (VFAAC)** was formed to assist referral to physicians experienced with valley fever

- **Arizona Department of Health Services**
  150 North 18th Avenue
  Phoenix, Arizona 85007
  Ph: (602) 364-3676
  Fax: (602)364-3199

- **Arizona Victims of Valley Fever**:
  www.arizonavictimsofvalleyfever.org

- **Craig Rundbaken, D.O. Respiratory and Valley Fever Clinic
  Contact information: AIRMEDVFC.COM
  and 623-975-0500**

- **Janice Blair, M.D.** of the Mayo Clinic of Scottsdale Arizona **www.mayoclinic.org**

- **Valley Fever America Foundation**: **www.valleyfever.com**

- **Garry Cole Ph.D.,** valley fever vaccine research; Department of Biology, The University of Texas, San Antonio: garry.cole@utsa.edu

GLOSSARY

A

acute
Having sudden onset, sharp rise and short course.

adenopathy
Enlargement of lymph nodes.

adjuvant
In immunology refers to a chemical added to an antigen to increase the immune response.

antibodies
Any of a large number of proteins of high molecular weight that are produced normally by specialized B-cells after stimulation by an antigen in an immune response typically consisting of four subunits including two heavy and two light chains also called immunoglobulins.

antifungal
Capable of neutralizing or eradicating fungus.

antigen
Any substance foreign to the body that evokes an immune response, either alone or often forming a complex with large molecular proteins and is capable of binding with a product of the immune receptors.

arthralgia
Pain in one or more joints.

arthroconidium
One of the small conidia born in chains by various fungi including genus Coccidioides.

arthrospore
The arthroconidia are arthrospores. The valley fever fungal spore.

azole
A class of antifungals used to treat Valley Fever (has a five member ring and contains at least one nitrogen)

B

B-cell lymphocytes
Any of the lymphocytes that have antigen binding antibody molecules on their surface that comprise the antibody secreting plasma cells. In mammals, differentiate in bone marrow when mature.

biosafety laboratory
Refers to the specifications and level of precaution mandated to prevent risk of infections. Four designations exist, a level requiring the highest mandate such as Ebola, Cocci is level 3 requirements.

bone scan

A nuclear medicine scan that uses radioactive chemicals to make images of bones and diseases of the bone. Commonly utilized for determining infections and cancer.

bronchoscope

Flexible instrument for inspecting bronchi. Can be utilized to take biopsies, lavage the airways for secretion and mucus analysis, and removal of foreign bodies.

C

cephalgia Headache.

cerebrospinal fluid A liquid fluid that is clear, colorless that bathes the brain and spinal cord.

chronic

A slow, progressive course of an illness of indefinite duration.

coccidioidal

Caused by the fungi of the genus Coccidioides.

coccidioidomycosis

A disease of humans and animals caused by the fungus of the genus Coccidioides immitis (C. immitis and C. posadasii) and marked especially by fever and pulmonary symptoms. Also known as San Joaquin Fever, San Joaquin Valley Fever, cocci, and Valley Fever.

cytokine
Any of a class of immunoregulatory proteins that are secreted by cells, especially of the immune system. They are known as cell communicators.

D

desert rheumatism
Infection with coccidioidomycosis associated with arthralgia and usually rash.

dimorphic
Occurring in two distinct forms.

disjunctor
In our context refers to a separation of arthrospores by connecting tissue when disturbed or disarticulated can propel through the atmosphere

disseminated
Widely dispersed in a tissue, organ, or entire body. In our context, refers to extra-pulmonary disease when the coccidioidomycosis travels to other organs usually via the circulation (hematogenous or lymphatic system).

E

EIA (enzyme immune assay)
One of several laboratory tests that measure antibodies.

embryo
Prenatal development between fertilized ovum and fetus.

embryogenic
The growth and development of an embryo.

empyema
Pus in the pleural space cavity in the chest but outside the lung.

endemic
Restricted or particular to a locality or region.

endospore
An asexual spore developed within the cell.

eosinophilia
An abnormal increased number of eosinophils in the blood that is characteristic of allergic states. Can also be seen with some infections, pneumonias and malignancies.

epidemic
A disease attacking many in a community simultaneously.

epidemiology
A branch of medical science that deals with the incidents, distribution and control of diseases in a population.

erythema multiforme
A skin disease characterized by a popular or vesicular lesion and reddening or discoloration of the skin in concentric zones about the lesion.

erythema nodosum

A skin condition characterized by small, tender reddened nodules under the skin as over the shin bones. Often accompanied by fever and transitory arthritic pain. Commonly considered a manifestation of hypersensitivity.

erythrocyte sedimentation rate

A blood test that correlates with inflammation (nonspecific).

fomites

An inanimate object (car, toy, door knobs, etc.) that may be contaminated with infectious organisms and serve in their transmission.

genus

A class, kind, group of species marked by common characteristics, alike in their broad features of their organization but different in detail.

granuloma

A mass or nodule of chronically inflamed tissue with granulation that is usually associated with the infective process.

haboob

Intense dust storm associated with wind, rain and thunderstorms carried on atmospheric gravity current.

hematogenous

Pertaining to anything produced from, derived from, or

transported by the blood. - Stedman's Medical Dictionary 24th Edition

histopathology
The microscopic study of diseased tissue

host
A living animal or plant in which the organism lives.

hydrocephalus
A condition marked by excessive accumulation of fluid dilating the cerebral ventricles, thinning the brain and causing separation of cranial bones.

hyphae
One of the threads that make up the mycelium of the fungus.

hypogylcorrhachia
A decrease concentration of glucose in the cerebrospinal fluid

immunodiffusion
A technique for obtaining a precipitant between an antibody and its specific antigen by suspending one in gel and letting the other migrate or by letting both antigen and antibody migrate through the gel.

incubation period
The period between the infection of an individual by

a pathogen and the manifestation of the disease that it causes (when the symptoms start).

lower life zone
The arid climate of the Southwest that is endemic for the fungal organism coccidioidomycosis.

lung cavity
An unfilled space within a mass in the lung.

lung nodule
A small mass, may be associated with infection.

lymph
Usually clear fluid that passes intercellular spaces of the body tissue into the lymphatic vessels and discharge into the blood by the thoracic duct. Lymph contains white blood cells and lymphocytes.

lymphatic
Pertaining to lymph, a vascular channel that transports lymph or a lymph node.

lymphocyte
Any of the colorless, weakly motile cells that originate from the stem cells and differentiate in lymphoid tissue (thymus or bone marrow). Includes cell mediators of immunity.

malignant
A tumor that is cancerous as opposed to benign.

mediastinum
The space in the chest between the pleural sacs of the lungs that contain all of the viscera of the chest except the lungs and the pleura.

meningitis
Inflammation of the meninges. May be associated with fever, malaise, vomiting and stiff neck.

micron
A unit length equal to one millionth of a meter. Also known as micrometer.

monsoon
Wind and rain storms caused by the seasonal changes in temperature over land and sea.

morphology
The form and structure of an organism or any of its parts.

myalgia
Pain in one or more muscles.

mycelium
The mass of interwoven filamentous hyphae that forms especially the vegetative body of a fungus and is submerged in another body (as of the soil or organic matter or tissue of the host).

mycology
The branch of biology dealing with fungi and fungal life.

mycosis

A disease caused by a fungus.

needle biopsy

Inserting a hollow needle through the skin and withdrawing the sample from the tissue or organ to examine it.

orphan disease

A disease which affects a relatively small number of individuals for which no drug therapy has been developed because of the small market. It would make the research and drug unprofitable.

pathogen

A microorganism that can cause disease (virus, fungus or bacteria).

PET scan

Positron emission tomography. Medical imaging using radionuclides to assess metabolism of tissue and abnormal findings. Increase metabolic uptake is seen with malignancy and infection.

phagocytosis

The engulfing and usually the destruction of particulate matter by phagocytes that serves an important bodily defense mechanism against infecting microorganisms.

plasma
The fluid part of the blood lymph that is distinguished from suspended material.

pleura
The lining of the lungs inner sac (visceral pleura) and outer sac (parietal pleura).

pleural effusion
An exudate of fluid from blood or lymph into the pleural cavity. Can occur with congestive heart failure, pneumonias and malignancies.

pleurisy
Inflammation of the pleura characterized by sudden onset of pain and difficulty breathing.

pneumonia
A disease of the lungs that is characterized especially by inflammation and consolidation of lung tissue followed by resolution. It is accompanied by fevers, chills, cough and difficulty breathing.

pneumothorax
A collection of air or gas in the pleural cavity, lung collapse.

Polymerase chain reaction (PCR)
A process that permits making, in the laboratory, unlimited numbers of copies of genes. This begins with a single molecule of genetic material, DNA.

Pregnancy Categories
A - Medication for which no harm has been demonstrated in a well designed study of pregnant and lactating women

Pregnancy Categories
B - Medication without known risk when used in human pregnancy or breastfeeding.

Pregnancy Categories
C - Medication whose use in human pregnancy or breastfeeding has not been adequately studied; risk of usage cannot be excluded but has not been proven.

Pregnancy Categories
D - Medication known to cause fetal harm when administered during pregnancy or infant breastfeeding

Pregnancy Categories
X - Medication judged to be unsafe (contraindicated) in pregnancy. Evidence of risk has accrued from clinical trials or post marketing surveillance.

Pyopneumothorax
A lung cavity rupture into pleural space. Lung collapse and pleural fluid accumulation can occur.

rheumatism
Any of the various conditions characterized by inflammation or pain in muscles, joints or fibrous tissue.

serology
A medical science dealing with blood serum and the immunologic reaction and properties.

serum
The watery portion of blood after coagulation-contains antibodies against specific organisms.

spore
A primitive, usually unicellular, environmentally resistant, dormant or reproductive body produced by plants, fungi, and some microorganisms. Capable of developing into a new individual either directly or after fusion with another spore.

stem cell
An unspecialized cell that gives rise to differentiated cells.

T-cell
Any of several lymphocytes (as a helper T-cell) that differentiate in the thymus, possesses highly specific cell surface antigen receptors. Note: T-cells are very important in fighting cocci.

Teratogenic
Causing abnormal development of the embryo.

titers
Strength of a solution or concentration of a substance in solution as determined by titration. (Loss in strength with greater dilution) In our context, high titers typical-

ly represent a worse case and higher risk of extra-pulmonary disease and lower titers represent less severe disease or resolving infection.

triazole
Newer antifungal medication such as itraconazole and fluconazole for treating fungal disease. Characterized by a ring compound composed of two carbon atoms and three nitrogen atoms.

Valley Fever
The term used for the constellation of signs and symptoms associated with coccidioidomycosis.

viscera
An internal organ of the body (heart, liver, intestine) located in large cavities of the trunk.

Sources:
Steadman's Medical Dictionary
Taber's Cyclopedic Medical Dictionary 22nd edition

BIBLIOGRAPHY

(n.d.). Retrieved from Arizona Department of Public Health: www.azdhs.gov

(n.d.). Retrieved from Valley Fever Center of Excellence: www.vfce.arizona.edu

(n.d.). Retrieved from Physicians' Desk Reference: **www.pdr.net**

Aleck K, Bartley D. (1997). Multiple malformation syndrome following fluconazole use in pregnancy. Report of an additional patient. American Journal of Medical Genetics, 72, 253-256.

Ampel NM, Dols CL, Galgiani JN. (1993). Coccidioidomycosis during human immune deficiency virus infection. Results of a prospective study in a coccidioidal endemic area. Am J Med, 94, 235-240.

Ampel, N. (1992, Jan-Feb). Coccidioidomycosis in the HIV-infected patient, diagnosis and treatment. AIDS Reader, 12-15.

Amphotericin B lipid complex in the treatment of invasive fungal infections. (2005). Clinical Infectious Disease Journal, 40 (6), 379-421.

Anti TNF-Drugs. (n.d.). (American College of Rheumatology) Retrieved from www.rheumatology.org

Biosafety and Microbiologic and biomedical laboratories. (n.d.). Retrieved from BMBL (5th edition): www.cdc.gov/biosafety/publication/bmb15/

Blair JE, Mayer AP, Currier J, Files JA, Nu Q. (2008). Coccidioidomycosis in elderly persons. Clinical Infectious Disease, 47 (12), 1513-1518.

Brown J, Benedict K, Park BJ, Thompson III, GR. (2013). Coccidioidomycosis: Epidemiology. Clinical Epidemiology, 5, pp. 185-197.

California department of public health. Coccidioidomycosis yearly summary report 2001 – 2010. Center for infectious disease, division of communicable disease control, infectious disease branch, surveillance and statistics section.

Clemens C, Laborn RL, Stephens D. (2006). Coccidioidomycosis, 6th International Symposium. Annals of New York Academy of Science, 1111.

Coccidioidomycosis – associated hospitalizations, California, USA 2000-2011. (2013). CDC, 19 (10).

Coccidioidomycosis in workers at an archaeological site – Dinosaur National Monument, Utah, June-July 2001. (2001, Nov 16). US Department of Health and Human Services, 50 (45).

Cole GT, Sun SH. (1985). Arthroconidium-spherule-endospore transformation in Coccidioides Immitis. (H. L. IN: Szaniszlo PG, Ed.) Fungal dimorphism: With emphasis on fungi pathogenic for humans, 281-233.

Colivas KN, Comrie DC. (2003). Modeling Valley Fever (Coccidioidomycosis) incidents on the basis of climate conditions. INT J Bio Meteorol, 47 (2), 87-101.

Comrie, A. (2005). Climate factors influencing Coccidioidomycosis seasonality and outbreaks. Environmental Health Perspective, 113, 688-692.

Convers, J. (1957). Effects of surface active antigens on endosporiolation of Coccidioides Immitis in a chemically defined medium. J Bacteriol, 74, 106-107.

Cortez KG, Walsh TJ, Bennett JE. (2003). Successful treatment of coccidioidal meningitis with Voriconazole. Clin Infect Dis, 15 (12), 1619-22.

Cox RA, Magee DM. (2004). Coccidioidomycosis: Host response and vaccine development. Clinical and Microbiology Review, 17 (4), 804-839.

Crum N, Lamb C, Utz G, Amundson D, Wallace M. (2002). Coccidioidomycosis outbreak among United States. The Journal of Infectious Disease, 186, pp. 865-868.

Crum NF, Ballond-Landa G. (2006). Coccidioidomycosis and pregnancy, case report and review of literature. American Journal of Medicine, 119 (993), e11-993, e17.

Deresinski, S. (1980). History of Coccidioidomycosis:

Dusk to dusk IM. (D. Stevens, Ed.) Coccidioidomycosis, 1-20.

Dismukes WE, Pappas PG, Sobel JD. (2003). Chapter 20 by Ampel, NM. In P. P. Dismukes WE, Clinical Mycology (pp. 331-327). Oxford University Press.

Drutz DJ, Catanzaro A. (1978). Coccidioidomycosis Part 1. AM Rev Respir Dis, 117, 559-585.

Drutz DJ, Catanzaro A. (1978). Coccidioidomycosis Part 2. Am Rev Resp. Dis, 117, 727-71.

Edwards PQ, Palmer CE. (1957). Prevalence and sensitivity to coccidioidin, with special reference to specific and non-specific reactions to coccidioidin and to histoplasmin. Dis Chest, 31, 35-60.

Fierer J, Waters C, Walls L. (2006). Both CD4+ and CD8+ T-cells can mediate vaccine-induced protection against Coccidioides Immitis infection in mice. Journal of Infectious Disease, 193, 1323-1331.

Fiese, M. (1958). Coccidioidomycosis. (C. C. Thomas, Ed.)

Fisher MC, Koenig GL, White TJ, Taylor JW. (2002). Molecular and phenotypic description of Coccioides Posadasii SP Nov, previously recognized as the non-California population of Coccioides Immitis. Mycologia, 94, 73-84.

Freedman SI, Ang EP, Halle RS. (1986). Identification of Cocci of the lung by fine needle aspiration biopsy.

ACTA Cytol, 30, 420-424.

Gadkowski, B and Stout, J. Clin Microbiol Rev April 2008, vol. 21, no. 2, 305-333.

Gaggo S, Buitrago MJ, Clemons KV, Cuenca-Estrella M, Mirels LF, Stevens DA. (2014, Feb). Development and validation of quantitative real time PCR assay for the early diagnosis of Coccidioidomycosis. Diagn Microbio Infect Dis.

Gaidici A, Saubolle MA. (2009). Transmission of Coccidia to human via a cat bite. J Clin Micro Biol, 47 (2), 505-506.

Galgiani J, Cantazaro A, Cloud G, et. al. (1993). Fluconazole therapy for coccidioidal meningitis. Annuals of Internal Medicine, 119 (1).

Galgiani JN, Ampel NM, Blair J, Catanzaro A, Johnson RH, Stevens DA, Williams PL. (2005). IDSA Guidelines, Coccidioidomycosis. In Clinical Infectious Diseases (Vol. 41, pp. 1217-1223).

Galgiani JN, Canetizara A, et al. (2000). Comparison of oral fluconazole and itraconazole for progressive non-meningeal coccidioidomycosis, a randomized double blind study. Annals of Internal Med, 133, 676-686.

Galgiani JN, Catanzaro A, Cloud GA, Higgs J, Friedman BA, Larson RA, Graybill JR. (1993). Niaid-Mycosis study group. Fluconazole therapy for coccidioidal meningitis. Annals of Internal Medicine, 119 (1).

Galgiani JN, et al. Coccidioidomycosis tutorial for primary care physicians. Valley Fever Center of Excellence. Tucson: University of Arizona.

Galgiani, J. (1999, Feb 16). Coccidioidomycosis: A regional disease of national importance, an update. Rethinking. Annals of Internal Medicine, 130 (4).

Galgiani, J. (1999, Feb 16). Coccidioidomycosis: A regional disease of national importance. Rethinking approach for. Annals of Internal Medicine, 130 (4), p. Part 1.

Gifford MA, Bus WC, Douds RJ, et al. (1936). Data on coccidioides fungus infection, Curran County Dept of Public Health. Ann Rep, 39-54.

Hedges E, Miller S. (1990, May). Coccidioidomycosis: Office Diagnosis and Treatment. American Family Practice, pp. 1499-1506.

Herr RA, Hung CY, Cole GT. (2007, Dec). Evaluation of two homologous Proline Rich proteins of Coccidioides Posadasii as candidate vaccines against coccidioidomycosis. Infecion and Immunity, 5777-5787.

Hospenthal, D. (2013, Sep 13). Coccidioidomycosis. Medline Reference Review.

Huang JY, Bristow B, Shafir S, Sorvillo F. (2012). Coccidioidomycosis – associated deaths, United States, 1990-2008. Emerging Infectious Disease, 18 (11).

Hyde, L. (1968). Coccidioidal pulmonary cavidation. 54 (Suppl 1), 273-277.

Hydrocephalus in Cocci meningitis. Case report and review of literature. (2000). Neurosurgery, 47 (3).

Increase in reported coccidioidomycosis – United States 1998-2011. (2013). Morbidity and mortality weekly report, 62 (12), 217-221.

Jick, S. (1999). Pregnancy outcomes after maternal exposure to fluconazole. Pharmacotherapy, 19 (2), 221-222.

Jones J, Fleming PL, Ciesielski C, Hugh DJ, Kaplan JE, Ward JW. (1995). Coccidioidomycosis among persons with AIDS in the United States. Journal of Infectious Disease, 171, 961-966.

Kirkland TN, Fierer J. (1996, July-Sept). Coccidioidomycosis, a re-emerging infectious disease. Emerging Infectious Disease Journal, 3 (2).

Kolivras K, Comrie KN. (2003). Modeling Valley Fever (Coccidioidomycosis) incidents on the basis of climate conditions. International Journal of Biometeorology, 47 (2), 87.

Kuberski T, Herrig J, Pappagianis D. (2010). False-Positive IgM serology in coccidioidomycosis. General Clinial Microbiology, 48 (6), 2047-2049.

Laniado-Laborin, R. (2007). Expanding the understanding of epidemiology of Coccidioidomycosis in the western hemisphere. Ann NY Acad Sci, 1111, 19-34.

Leake JA, Mosley DG, England B, et. al. (2000). Risk factors for acute symptomatic Coccidioidomycosis among elderly persons in Arizona 1996-97. J infect Dis, 18 (4), 1435-1440.

Malo J, Lurashchi-Monjagatta C, Wolk DM, Thompson R, Hage C, Knox K. (n.d.). Update on the diagnosis of pulmonary Coccidioidomycosis.

Marshall JK, Irving EJ. (1997, Sept). Successful therapy of refractory erythema nodosum associated with Crohn's. Canada Journal of Gastroenterology, 11 (6).

Micrometics. (n.d.). Retrieved from www.micromedx.com

Miller DD, Cowen EW, Nguyen JC, et. al. (2010). Melanoma associated with long-term Voriconazole therapy. New manifestations of chronic photosensitivity. Arch Dermatol, 146 (3), 300-304.

Mira Vista Diagnostics. (n.d.). Indianapolis, IN.

Morice C, Archer A, Soufir N, Michel M, Comoz F, Leroy D, Verneuil L. (2010, 12 16). Multifocal aggressive squamous cell carcinomas induced by prolonged Voriconazole therapy: A case report. Retrieved from Case Rep Med 210:351084.

Morrow, W. (2006). Holocene Coccidioidomycosis: Valley Fever and early Holocene bison (Bison antiquus). Mycologia 98.5 669, 98 (5), 669-677.

Ophuls W, Moffitt HC. (1900). A new pathogenic

mold (formerly described as a protozoa: Coccidioides immitis pyogens): Preliminary report. Philidelphia Med J.S., 1471-1472.

Palmer CE, Edwards PQ, Alfather WE. (1957). Characteristics of skin reactions to coccidioidin and histoplasmin, with evidence of unidentified sources of sensitivity in some geographic areas (abstract). Symposium on Coccidioidomycosis, Communicable Disease Center, 575, 171-180.

Pappagianis D, Zimmer BL. (1990, July). Serology of coccidioidomycosis. Clinical Microbiology Reviews, 247-268.

Pappagianis, D. (2005, Apr 25). Application and interpretation of serologic tests. School of Medicine, University of California, Davis, Coccidioidomycosis serology laboratory, Davis.

Pappagianis, D. (1988). Epidemiology of Coccidioidomycosis. Curr Top Med Mycol, 2, 199-238.

Pappagianis, D. (1988). Epidimiology of Coccidioidomycosis infection. Curr Top Med Mycol, 2, 199-238.

Peterson CM, Schuppert K, Kelly PC, & Pappagianis D. (1993). Coccidioidomycosis and pregnancy. Obstetrical and Gynecologic Survey, 48 (3), 149-156.

Peterson LR, Marshall SL, Barton-Dixon C, Hajjeh RA, Lindsey MD, Warnock DW, et al. (2004, Apr). Coccidioidomycosis among workers at an archaeological site, Northeastern Utah. Journal of Emerging Infectious Disease, 10 (4).

Polidge CR, et al. (2006). Revisiting the sensitivity of serologic testing in culture-positive Coccidioidomycosis. Ann NY Acad Sci 2007, 1111, 301-314.

Posada, A. (1892). Un Nuevo Casa De Micosis Fungoiden Con Psorospermis. Ann Circulo Medico, 15, pp. 585-597.

Rixfort E, Gilchrist TC. (1896). Two cases of protozoan (coccidioidal) infections of the skin and other organs. Johns Hopkins Hospital, REP. 1, 209-268.

Rosenstein NE, Emery KW, Werner SB, et al. (2001). Risk factors for severe pulmonary and disseminated Coccidioidomycosis: Curran County, CA 1995-1996. Clin Infect Dis, 32 (5), 708-715.

Saubolle MA, McKellar PP, Sussland D. (2007). Epidemiologic, clinical, and diagnostic aspects of Coccidioidomycosis. J Clin Microbiol, 45 (1), 26-30.

Schneider E, Hajjeh R, Spiegel R, Jibson R, Harp E, Marshall G, et al. (1997, Mar 19). A Coccidioidomycosis outbreak following the 1994, Northridge, CA earthquake. Journal of the American Medical Association, 227 (AMA).

Smith CE, Beard RR. (1946a). Varieties of Coccidioidal infection in relation to the epidemiology and control of the disease. Am J Public Health, 36, 1394-1402.

Smith CE, Beard RR, Rosenberger HG, Whiting EG. (1946). Effective season and dust control on coccidioidomycosis. J AM Med Assoc, 132, 833-838.

Smith CE, Salto MT, Simons SA. (1956). Patterns of 39,500 serological tests in Coccidioidomycosis. JAMA, 160, 546-552.

Smith CE, Whiting EG, Baker EE, Rosenberger HG, Beard RR, Saito MT. (1948). The use of coccidioidin. AM Rev Tuberc, 57, 330-360.

Smith, C. (1951). Diagnosis of pulmonary coccidioidal infection in California medicine. 75, 385-391.

Sobonya R, Barbee RA, Wiens J, Trego D. (1990). Detection of fungi and other pathogens in immunocompromised patients by bronchoalveolar lavage in an area endemic of. Chest, 97 (6), 1349-1355.

Sobonya RE, Ynez J, Klotz SA. (2014). Cavitary pulmonary Coccidiodomycosis: Pathological and Clinical correlative disease. Hum Pathol, 45 (1), 153-159.

Stevens, D. (1995, Apr 20). Coccidioidomycosis, a review article. New England Journal of Medicine, 332 (16).

Successful therapy of refractory erythema nodosum with Crohn's disease using potassium iodide. (1997). Can J Gastroenteral, 11 (6).

Sun SH, Huppert M. (1976). A cytological study of morphogenesis in Coccidioides Immitis. Sabouraudia, 14, 185-198.

Sunenshine RH, Anderson, Erhort L, et al. (2007). Public Health Surveillance for Coccidioidomycosis in Arizona. Ann NY Acad Sci, 1111, 96-102.

Talamantes J, Behseta S, Zender CS. (2007). Fluctuations in climate and incidents of Coccidioidomycosis in Curran County, CA. A review. Ann NY Acad Science, 1111, 73-82.

Tamerius JD, Comrie DC. (2011). Coccidioidomycosis incidents in Arizona predicted by seasonal precipitation. PLOS 1, 6 (6), e21009.

Tierney LM Jr., Schwartz RA. (1984). Erythema Nodosum. American Family Physician, 30 (4), 227-32.

Tiphine M, Letscher-Bru V, Herbrecht R. (1999). Amphotericin B and its new formulations: Pharmacologic characteristics, clinical efficacy, and tolerability. Journal of transplant and infectious disease (Transpl Infect Dis), 1 (4), 273-283.

Tucker RM, Galgiani J, Denning DW, Hunson LH, et. al. (1990). Treatment of Coccidioidal meningitis with fluconazole. Reviews of Infectious Disease, 12 (Supp 3).

Tucker RM, Galgiani JN, Dennis DW, Hansen LH, Graybill JR, & Shark. (1999). Treatment of coccidioidal meningitis with fluconazole. Reviews of infectious disease, 12 (supp 3), s380-389.

Valdivia L, Nix D, Wright M, Lindberg E, Fagan T, Lieberman D, et al. (2006, June). Coccidioidomycosis as a common cause of community acquired pneumonia. Emerging Infectious Disease Journal, 12 (8).

Valley Fever of the San Joaquin Valley and the fungus Coccidioides. (1937). Cal West Medicine, 47 (3), 151-155.

Zonios DI, Bennett, JE. (2008). Update on azole antifungal therapy. Seminars in respiratory and critical care medicine, 29 (2), 198-2010.